Blythe/Pöldinger · German-English Glossary

German-English Glossary of Psychiatric Terms

G. BLYTHE
(English editor)

W. PÖLDINGER
(Psychiatric consultant)

URBAN & SCHWARZENBERG
München – Wien – Baltimore

English editor
George Blythe, Spechtstr. 3, CH-4106 Therwil BL

Psychiatric consultant
Prof. Dr. med Walter Pöldinger,
Psychiatrische Universitäts-Klinik, Wilhelm-Klein-Str. 27, CH-4025 Basel

Urban & Schwarzenberg
Pettenkoferstraße 18
D-8000 München 2
Germany

Urban & Schwarzenberg, Inc.
7 East Redwood Street
Baltimore, Maryland 21 202
USA

CIP-Kurztitelaufnahme der Deutschen Bibliothek

Blythe, George:
German-English Glossary of Psychiatric Terms/
G. Blythe (Engl. ed.). W. Pöldinger (Psychiatric consultant). –
München; Wien; Baltimore:
Urban und Schwarzenberg, 1987.
ISBN 3-541-70191-9 (München, Wien)
ISBN 0-8067-0191-0 (Baltimore)
NE: Pöldinger, Walter; HST

Printed in Germany. Wagner GmbH, Nördlingen

ISBN 3-541-70191-9 München
ISBN 0-8067-0191-9 Baltimore

Table of Contents

Introduction VII
Advice to the User X
Unchanged Loanwords XII
Abbreviations XIV
Bibliography XVII
Figures XVIII
Table XXVII
German-English Glossary 1
Appendix: A List of Lesser-Known Phobias 93

Inhaltsverzeichnis

Vorwort IX
Benutzerhinweise XI
Unveränderte Lehnwörter XIII
Abkürzungen XV
Literatur XVII
Abbildungen XIX
Tabelle XXVII
Deutsch-Englisches Glossar 1
Appendix: Verzeichnis wenigbekannter Phobien 93

Introduction

This glossary represents an initial attempt to equate some of the more important, elusive or problematic terms used in German and English texts on psychiatry and psychology. It is clear that a publication of this size cannot be fully comprehensive, since psychosomatic terminology alone passes through the interface of many disciplines. The aim is rather to provide a compact, quick reference for translating German texts on these and allied subjects into English or for German-speaking doctors wishing to publish papers in English.

At this writing no German-English dictionary is available on psychiatry or psychology, which is regrettable considering how the two languages have enriched one another in these fields. For this reason the glossary will concentrate more on the mental aspects than on, say, drug therapy, which is already covered by available medical and pharmaceutical bilingual dictionaries.

Brief definitions are provided where appropriate or possible. These are intended only as a guide since they do not always concur totally in the two languages, and may even vary from specialist to specialist. Indeed, one of the problems of terminology in this whole field is that it is not always immediately apparent from which language certain concepts stem or which school should be credited with the authentic definition. It is fairly clear that *abreaction* is a translation of the German *Abreagieren,* but it is not so apparent with *acting out (agieren),* while the parentage and interpretation of *Präsentiersymptom* is very dubious. This is hardly surprising when one considers that leading authors such as Alexander have worked and published in both Germany and in the United States. Similarly, Sifneos defined 'affect', 'emotion' and 'feeling'. But whether his distinctions will be accepted by other writers of English, or be followed by German-speaking authors, is a matter for speculation.

These simple examples will illustrate some of the difficulties of trying to bring the terms used in both languages into alignment. They also probably explain the lack of bilingual reference works in this field.

A good part of the glossary was compiled in the course of revising a series of editions of 'Psychosomatic Disorders in General Practice' by B. Luban-Plozza and W. Pöldinger.

This small work may fill some of the lacunae in available literature, but it will of course never replace *Fingerspitzengefühl* – which is an important part of psychiatry itself!

George Blythe

Acknowledgments

The authors would like to thank colleagues in medical and linguistic fields who gave advice on some of the entries or provided additional literature.
Professor R. R. Tilleard-Cole, Oxford University; Dr A. Baines, Canterbury. Members of F. Hoffmann-La Roche, Basel: Frau R. Pötzsch, Herr J.-P. Geri, Dr J. Haller, Professor M. Klingler, Mr J. W. Parry, Professor E. C. Senay, Mr J. Ward. Sandoz, Basel: Mr S. Cooper, Dr C. Weil.

Special mention must be made of the excellent works of reference *The Longman Dictionary of Psychology and Psychiatry* and the *Oxford Textbook of Psychiatry,* from which some of the definitions and terms in this glossary were abstracted in cases where they agreed essentially with the German terms. The reader desirous of studying the terms purely in English and in greater detail would be well advised to consult these works.

Further help, particularly in simplifying the definitions, was obtained from the *Encyclopaedia of Psychiatry for General Practitioners* published by Roche Products Ltd., England.

The appendix on phobias has been modified from a table appearing in a Sandoz (Basle) publication (*Common Psychiatric Terms in 4 Languages*, 1972) and in the *Glossaire de Psychiatrie* by P. Marchais. Masson & Cie, Paris, 1970.

Vorwort

Das vorliegende Glossar verdankt seine Entstehung der Übersetzung des Buches *Der psychosomatisch Kranke in der Praxis* von B. Luban-Plozza und W. Pöldinger vom Deutschen ins Englische. Bei diesen Übersetzungsarbeiten hat es sich gezeigt, wie schwierig es ist, bestimmte Fachausdrücke aus dem Bereich der Psychosomatik und Psychoanalyse, aber auch der allgemeinen Psychiatrie, vom Deutschen ins Englische und umgekehrt zu übertragen. Eine Analyse dieser Schwierigkeiten hat ergeben, daß vielfach in dem jeweiligen Sprachraum bestimmte Fachausdrücke in unterschiedlicher Bedeutung gebraucht werden.

Herr Blythe als Übersetzer hat sich nun der Mühe unterzogen, durch den Vergleich verschiedener Fachwörterbücher, den Vergleich von Übersetzungen mit dem jeweiligen Original und durch persönlichen Kontakt mit vielen Autoren der schwierigen Frage nachzugehen, wie und unter welchen Bedingungen bestimmte Fachausdrücke am besten in die jeweils andere Sprache zu übersetzen sind. Außerdem hat Herr Blythe sich bei seinen Recherchen bemüht, die Auffassungen verschiedener Autoren zu ergründen.

Wie notwendig diese Arbeit gewesen ist, hat der Vergleich verschiedener Übersetzungen gezeigt. Wir mußten feststellen, daß oft durch die alleinige wörtliche Übersetzung bestimmter Sätze der Sinn entstellt wurde und somit der Zusammenhang vollkommen verloren gegangen ist. Während der Stunden gemeinsamer Diskussion mit Herrn Blythe habe ich nämlich nicht nur die Präzisierung von englischen Übersetzungen gelernt, sondern mir ist auch klar geworden, daß wir oft gewisse Fachausdrücke in der eigenen Sprache verwenden, ohne zu berücksichtigen, welche verschiedenen Bedeutungsinhalte sie haben können. Es ist deshalb ein Anliegen dieses Buches, eine erste Ordnung in die Begriffvielfalt zu bringen. So habe ich den Wunsch, daß dieses Wörterbuch all jenen von Nutzen sein wird, die sich in die englischsprachige Literatur dieses Fachgebietes vertiefen oder selbst übersetzen.

Ganz besonders herzlich möchte ich mich bei Herrn Blythe für seine Mühe und Akribie bedanken; Dank auch dem Verlag und seinen Mitarbeitern für die gute Zusammenarbeit.

Basel, im Frühjahr 1986 *W. Pöldinger*

Advice to the User

The terms selected for this glossary are those likely to present problems, no matter how small, to a varied readership. DSM-III terms (see Abbreviations, p. XV), which are restricted to mental disease, have been kept to a minimum, since an extensive listing in the two languages is already available. Most of the DSM-III terms are in any case translated rather literally. This glossary includes therapies, psychological phenomena, psychoanalytical principles, and some other terms encountered in psychiatry and psychosomatic medicine. Where several terms are given as possible translations, the first listed are either preferable or more common unless otherwise stated. Frequently cited sources are listed in the bibliography and referred to by numbers in brackets when quoted.

German entry headwords are listed, with few exceptions, in their natural, noninverted word order, since it is frequently the adjectives that constitute difficulties for the translator in this field.

Ample cross-references based on nouns are also provided.

For the convenience particularly of the user unfamiliar with German alphabetization rules, the entries have otherwise been ordered according to English-language convention: The umlaut letters ä, ö, and ü have been written as such (not as ae, oe or ue), but the umlaut ignored in alphabetic order, and the German letter ß has been written as ss throughout. Capitalization of German expressions follows German rules, i. e. nouns are capitalized, whereas other parts of speech are not.

The abridged definitions given in English represent in some cases a compromise between different schools or between German and English standpoints. They are not intended to be textbook material but merely a guide so that the translator or author knows he is 'on the right track' in choosing an expression.

In the course of time it is inevitable that gaps will be revealed in a pioneer work of this type, and suggestions or criticisms are invited from users for correction in later editions. The bibliography given provides further useful information in the matter of definitions dealt with separately in the two languages.

Benutzerhinweise

Die ausgewählten Stichworte sind überwiegend solche Begriffe, die für eine breit gefächerte Leserschaft mehr oder weniger problematisch sind. Die DMS-III Begriffe, die auf Geisteskrankheiten beschränkt sind, sind auf einer möglichst geringen Anzahl gehalten, da in beiden Sprachen bereits ausführliche Auflistungen erhältlich sind. Die meisten DMS-III Begriffe sind ohnehin ziemlich wörtlich übersetzt worden. Dieses Glossar berücksichtigt darüber hinaus Behandlungsmethoden, psychologische Phänomene, psychoanalytische Grundsätze und einige andere Begriffe, auf die man in Psychiatrie und psychosomatischer Medizin stößt. Wo mehrere Begriffe als mögliche Übersetzung aufgeführt sind, ist der zuerst Genannte entweder vorzuziehen oder der gebräuchlichere, falls nicht anders vermerkt.

Zusammengesetzte deutsche Hauptstichwörter sind bis auf wenige Ausnahmen in unveränderter Reihenfolge aufgeführt, da es regelmäßig die Adjektive sind, die dem Übersetzer auf diesem Gebiet Schwierigkeiten bereiten.

Zahlreiche Kreuzverweise, größtenteils auf der Basis von Substantiven, mögen die Auffindbarkeit der Stichwörter erleichtern.

Um dem mit den deutschen Alphabetisierungsregeln nicht vertrauten Leser entgegenzukommen, sind die Stichwörter nach den Regeln aufgereiht, wie sie im englischen Sprachraum üblich sind: Die Buchstaben ä, ö und ü sind zwar in dieser Form erhalten, jedoch ohne Rücksicht auf den Umlaut wie a, o bzw. u eingeordnet. Der Buchstabe ß erscheint durchweg als ss.

Die verkürzten Definitionen auf englisch stellen in manchen Fällen Kompromisse dar zwischen verschiedenen Schulen oder zwischen deutschen und englischen Standpunkten. Sie sollen kein Lehrbuchmaterial sein, sondern nur Hinweis, damit der Übersetzer oder Autor sich auf der richtigen Spur bei der Wahl eines Begriffes weiß.

Im Laufe der Zeit wird es unvermeidlich sein, daß sich in einer Pionierarbeit dieser Art Lücken auftun werden, und Vorschläge oder Kritik der Benutzer sind für die Verbesserung späterer Ausgaben sehr willkommen. Die vorliegende Bibliographie enthält weitere nützliche Information über die aufgeführten Definitionen in der einen oder der anderen Sprache.

Unchanged Loanwords

The difficulty of translating some words connected with this field is shown by the number of borrowed words that have not been thoroughly 'naturalized' in either language. A few examples are given below.

Examples of English words used in German

Compliance; α-up, β-down regulation; borderline; doctor shopping; dreamy state; flapping tremor; flush; intensive care syndrome; jet lag; knockout; open-door system; overprotection; trance; tranquilizer; trip; workaholic.

Examples of German words used in English

Anlage; Dasein (sometimes); Doppelgänger* (-erlebnis); Eigenwelt; Einstellung*; Einheitspsychose*; Ganzfeld; Gestalt; Kindergarten; Mitgehen*; Prägnanz* (principle of); Vorbeireden*; Wanderlust; Weltanschauung; Zeitgeist.

(Most of these expressions will be found uncapitalized in English texts.)

* Defined in the glossary.

Unveränderte Lehnwörter

Wie schwer es ist, einige Begriffe aus diesem Fachgebiet zu übersetzen, mag die große Zahl übernommener Ausdrücke verdeutlichen, die in der jeweiligen Fremdsprache noch nicht völlig aufgenommen worden sind.

Beispiele für englische Wörter, die Eingang in die deutsche Sprache gefunden haben

Compliance; α-up/β-down regulation; borderline; doctor shopping; dreamy state; flapping tremor; flush; intensive care syndrome; jet lag; knockout; open-door system; overprotection; trance; tranquilizer; trip; workaholic.

Beispiele für deutsche Wörter, die Eingang in die englische Sprache gefunden haben

Anlage; Dasein; Doppelgänger* (-erlebnis); Eigenwelt; Einstellung*; Einheitspsychose*; Ganzfeld; Gestalt; Kindergarten; Mitgehen*; Prägnanz* (-prinzip); Vorbeireden*; Wanderlust; Weltanschauung; Zeitgeist.

(In englischsprachigen Texten werden diese Wörter meistens klein geschrieben.)

---

* Im Glossar definiert.

Abbreviations

ICD	International Classification of Diseases. WHO, Geneva
DSM	Diagnostic and Statistical Manual of Mental Disorders, American Psychiatric Association
REM	Rapid Eye Movements
NREM	Non-Rapid-Eye Movements
U.K.	United Kingdom (British usage)
U.S.	United States (American usage)
→	see also
cf.	compare
Ref.	Source or recommended further reading. See also Bibliographie, p. XVII.

Abkürzungen

ICD	International Classification of Diseases. WHO, Geneva
DSM	Diagnostic and Statistical Manual of Mental Disorders, American Psychiatric Association
REM	Rapid Eye Movements
NREM	Non-Rapid-Eye Movements
U.K.	United Kingdom (britischer Ausdruck)
U.S.	United States (amerikanischer Ausdruck)
→	siehe
cf.	vergleiche
Ref.	weiterführender Literaturbeleg oder Quelle (Literaturverzeichnis S. XVII)

Bibliography
Literatur

1. Alexander, F. G., S. T. Selesnick: The History of Psychiatry. Harper and Row, New York 1968. (deutsche Ausgabe: Geschichte der Psychiatrie. Diana-Verlag, Zürich 1969)
2. Brill, A. A.: Basic Principles of Psychoanalysis. Washington Square Press, New York 1968.
3. Campbell, J. (ed.): The Portable Jung. Penguin, Harmondsworth, Middlesex 1982.
4. Common Psychiatric Terms in 4 Languages. Sandoz, Basle 1971.
5. Eaton, M. T., M. H. Peterson, T. A. Davis (eds.): Psychiatry: Medical Outline Series. Medical Examination Co., Garden City New York 1981. (deutsche Ausgabe: Hans Huber, Berne, Switzerland)
6. Gelder, M., D. Gath, R. Mayou: Oxford Textbook of Psychiatry. Oxford University Press, Oxford – New York – Toronto 1983.
7. Goldenson, R. M. (ed.): Longman Dictionary of Psychology and Psychiatry. Longman, New York – London 1984.
8. Leigh, D., C. M. B. Pare, J. Marks (eds.): Encyclopedia of Psychiatry for General Practitioners. Roche Products Ltd., London 1972.
9. Mental Disorders: Classification in Accordance with ICD-9. World Health Organization, Geneva 1978.
10. Neel, A. F.: a) Theories of Psychology: A Handbook. Schenkmann Publishing Company, Cambridge, Mass. 1969. b) Handbuch der psychologischen Theorien. Kindler, München 1974.
11. Peters, U. H.: Wörterbuch der Psychiatrie und medizinischen Psychologie. Urban & Schwarzenberg, München – Wien – Baltimore 1984.

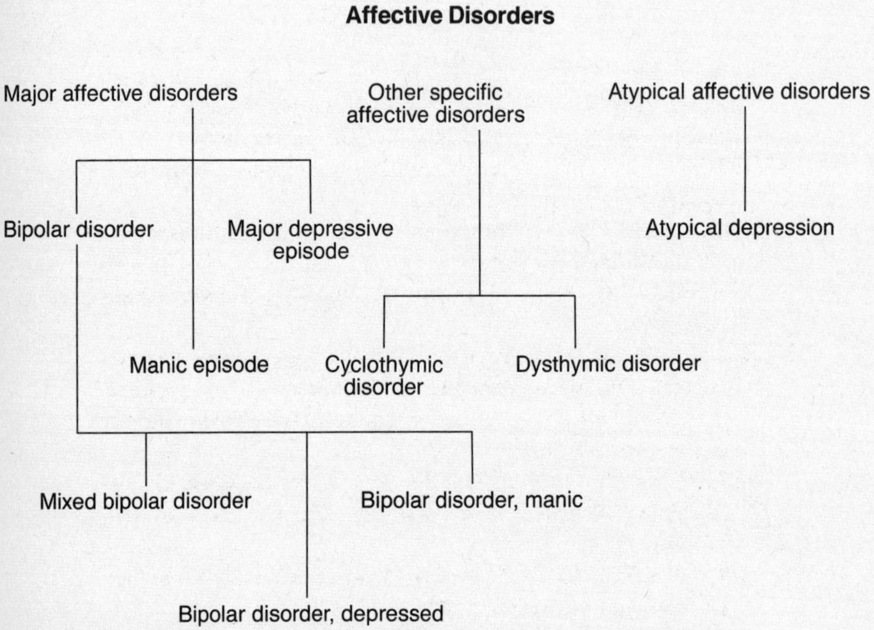

Fig. 1 Affective disorders (from Peters [12])

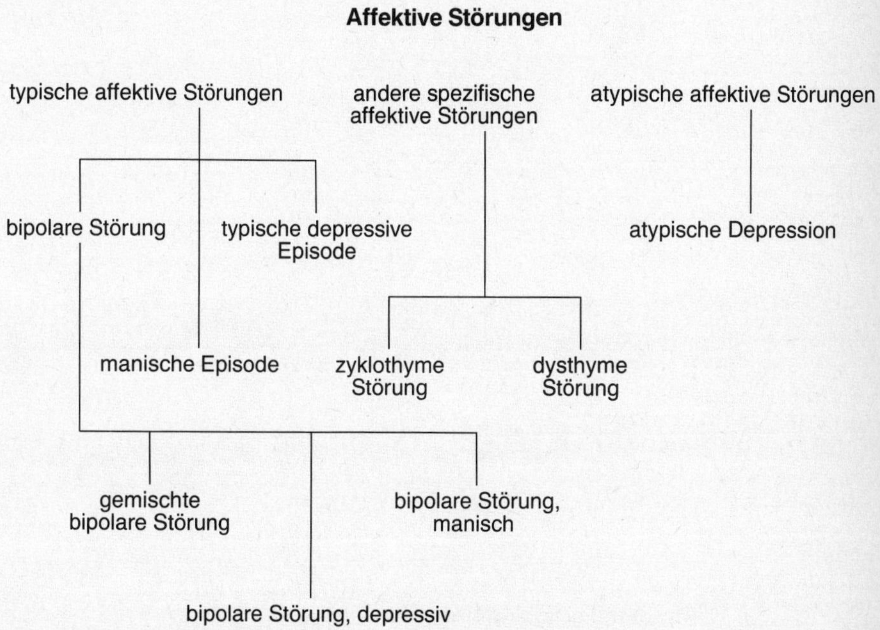

Abb. 1 Affektive Störungen (nach Peters [12])

Topographic model (systematic approach) showing levels of consciousness in psychoanalysis

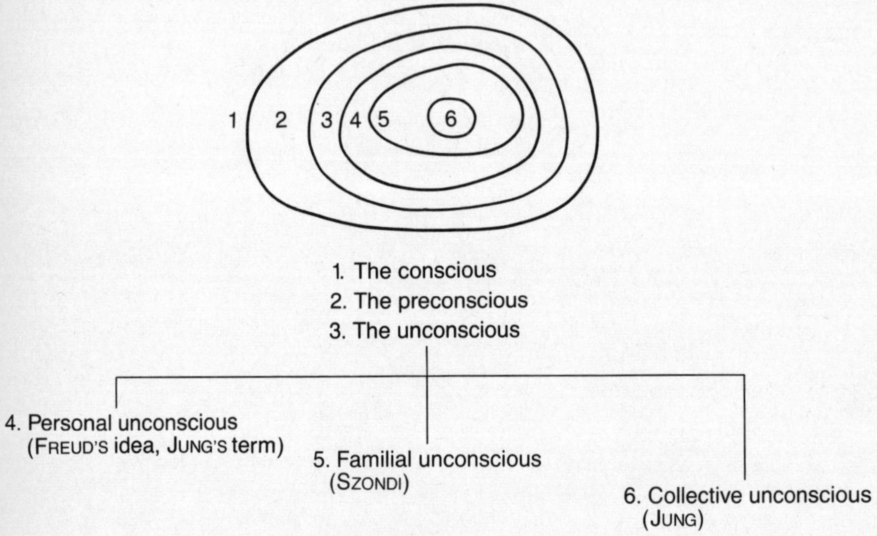

Structural model of the mind in psychoanalysis

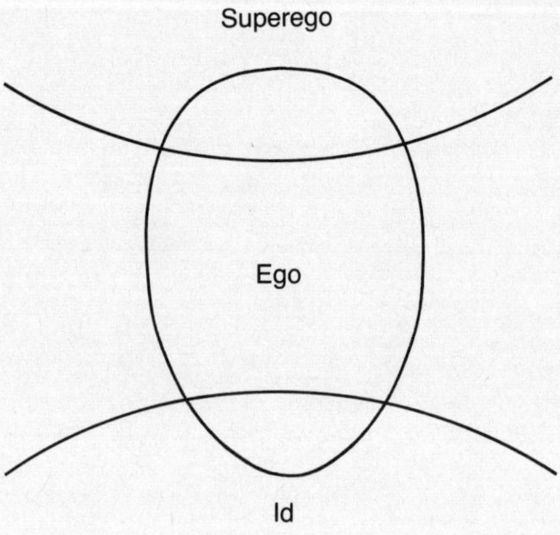

Fig. 2 Topographic and structural models in psychoanalysis

Topische Einteilung psychischer Gegebenheiten in der Psychoanalyse

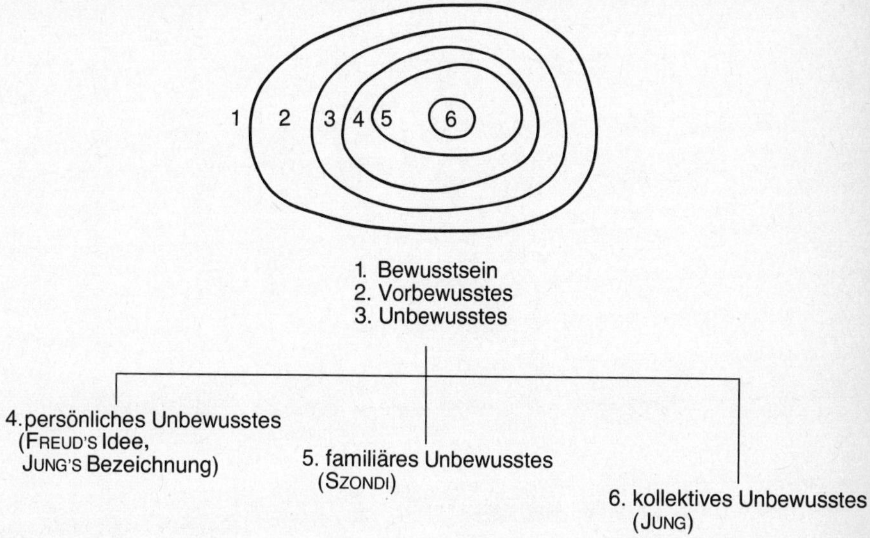

Strukturelle Einteilung der Seele in der Psychoanalyse

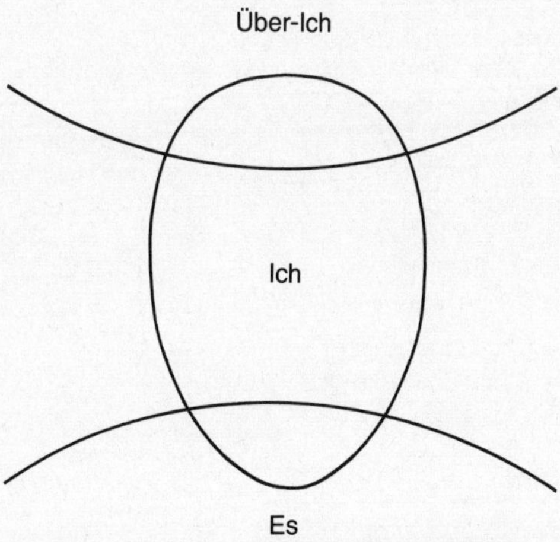

Abb. 2 Topische und strukturelle Einteilungen der Seele in der Psychoanalyse

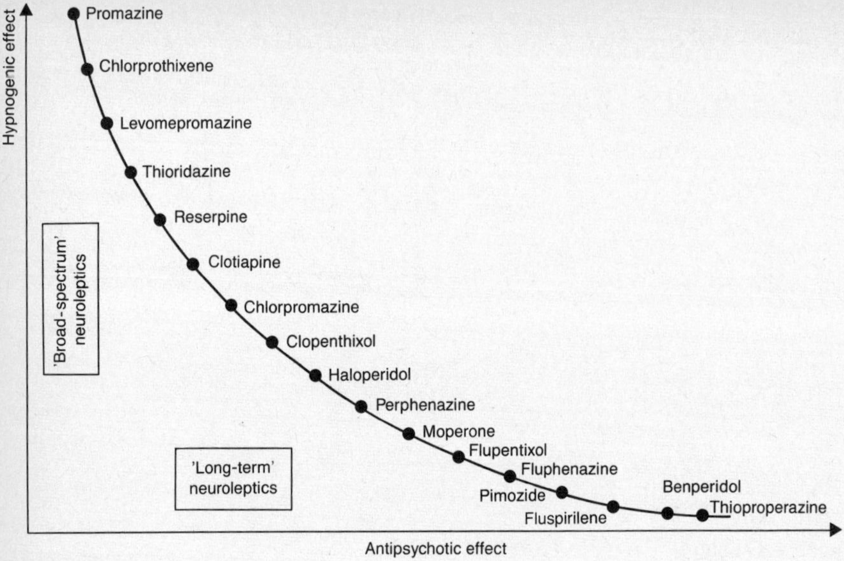

Fig. 3 Diagram of the properties of some neuroleptics.

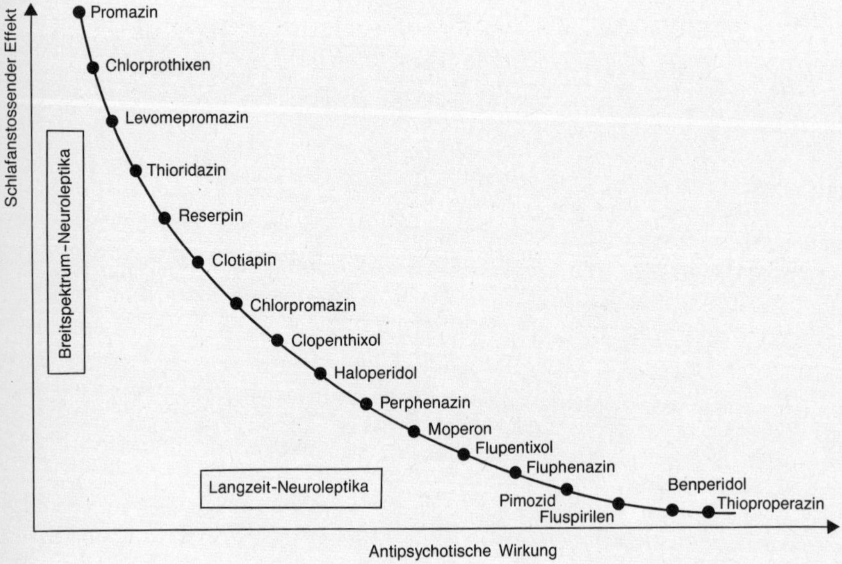

Abb. 3 Schematische Darstellung der Wirkungsqualitäten einiger Neuroleptika

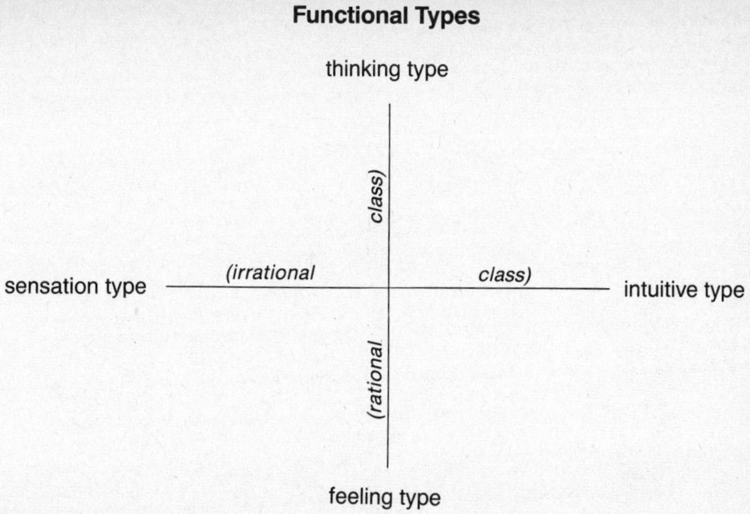

Fig. 4 Schematic representation of JUNG's functional types. All may be either extrovert or introvert (→ **extravertiert, introvertiert**)

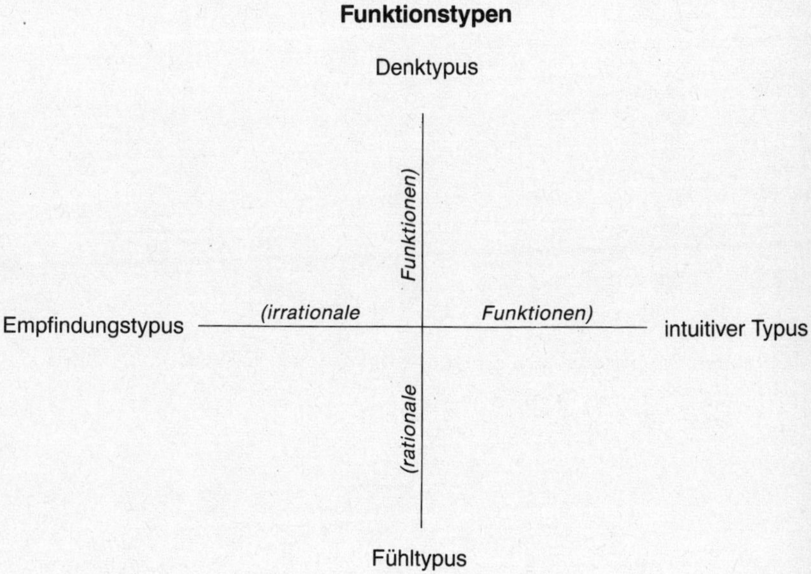

Abb. 4 Funktionstypen nach JUNG. Alle können → introvertiert oder → extravertiert sein (siehe Glossar).

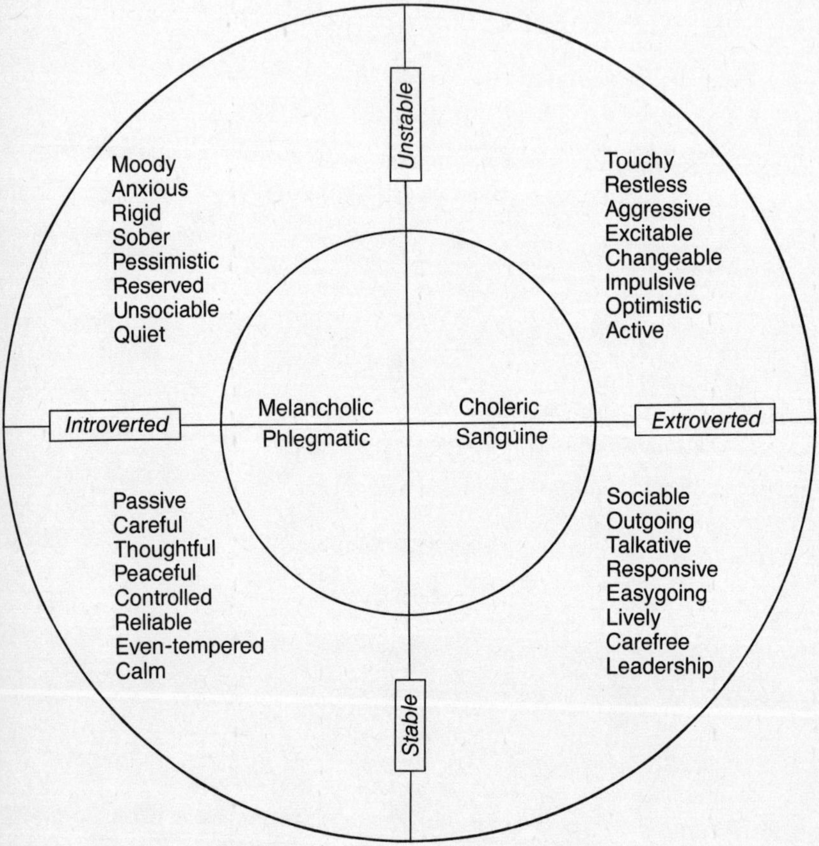

Fig. 5 Personality structure and correlated temperaments according to Eysenck (nach Eysenck, H. J.: The Dimensions of Personality. Routledge & Kegan, London 1947)

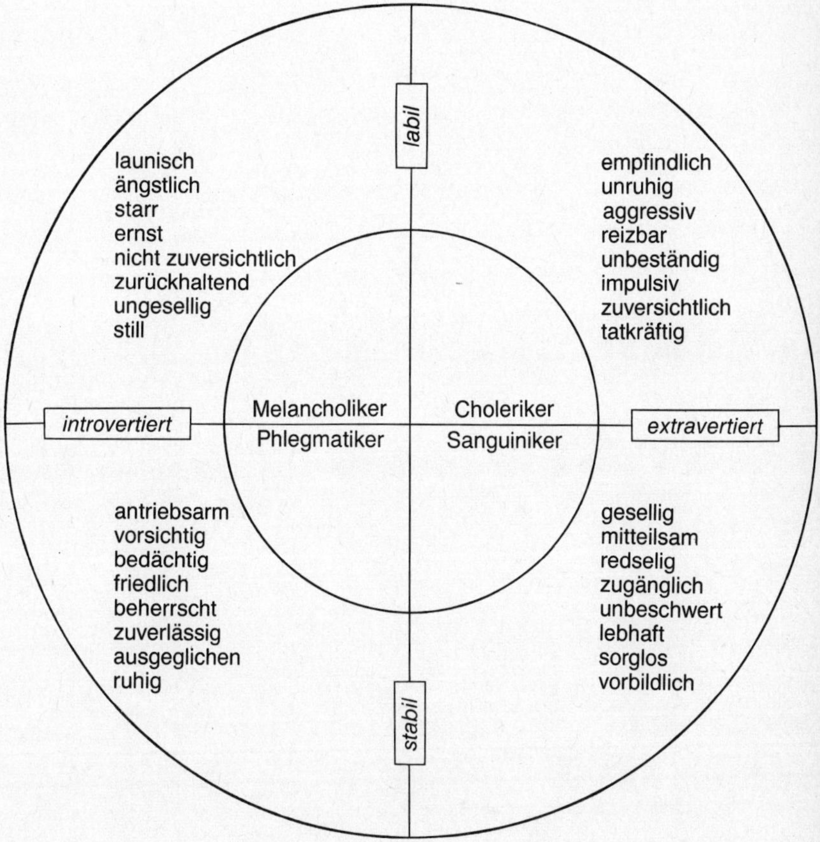

Fig. 5 Persönlichkeitsstruktur und zugehörige Temperamente (nach Eysenck, H. J.: The Dimensions of Personality. Routledge & Kegan, London 1947, zitiert und übersetzt in: Tilleard-Cole, R. R.: Persönlichkeitsaspekte im medizinischen Umgang. Hexagon „Roche" 6/4 [1978] 1–7).

Table 1 Neuroses. DSM-III does not include a formal category of neurosis – but instead divides them as follows (modified from the Oxford Textbook of Psychiatry [6], p. 135):

Affective disorders
300.40 Dysthymic disorder (depressive neurosis)

Anxiety disorders
300.21 Agoraphobia with panic attacks
300.22 Agoraphobia without panic attacks
300.23 Social phobia
300.01 Panic disorder
300.02 Generalized anxiety disorder
300.30 Obsessive compulsive disorder

Somatoform disorders
300.81 Somatization disorder
300.11 Conversion disorder
307.80 Psychogenic pain disorder
300.70 Hypochondriasis

Dissociative disorders
300.60 Depersonalization disorder

Tabelle 1 Neurosen. DSM-III sieht keine Kategorie der Neurosen vor, sondern teilt sie wie folgt ein (modifiziert nach *Oxford Textbook of Psychiatry* [6], S. 135):

Affektive Störungen
300.40 dysthyme Störung (oder depressive Neurose)

Angstsyndrome
300.21 Agoraphobie mit Panikattacken
300.22 Agoraphobie ohne Panikattacken
300.23 soziale Phobie
300.01 Paniksyndrom
300.02 generalisiertes Angstsyndrom
300.30 Zwangssyndrom (Zwangsneurose)

Somatoforme Störungen
300.81 Somatisierungssyndrom
300.11 Konversionssyndrom (hysterische Neurose, Konversionstyp)
307.80 psychogenes Schmerzsyndrom
300.70 Hypochondrie (hypochondrische Neurose)

Dissoziative Störungen (hysterische Neurosen, dissoziative Form)
300.60 Depersonalisationssyndrom (oder Depersonalisationsneurose)

A

Abfuhr discharge; release.
Discharge is used when there is an abrupt reduction in psychic tension. This may be brought about by dreaming, fantasizing or symptomatic acts. *Release* refers more to the effect produced by rational working-through, e.g. in coping mechanisms for anxiety.
Caveat: Discharge procedure is the process of discharging a patient from the hospital **(Entlassung).** Depending on the context, there are many other ways of translating **Abfuhr:** removal, disposal, rebuff. **Jemandem eine Abfuhr erteilen** to rebuff; to give someone the brush-off.
Abführmittel laxative, purgative.

Abhängigkeit dependency; dependence.
A state in which all types of assistance and guidance may be sought or expected. In psychoanalysis its origins are considered to be in the oral stage of infant development. Not to be confused with *psychological dependence* which is dependence on psychoactive substances where withdrawal symptoms are milder than in true addiction.
→ **Sucht**, → **Suchtstoffabhängigkeit**, → **Zweizügelabhängigkeit**.

abreagieren to abreact.
To release a repressed emotion, in the sense that painful experiences which had been buried in the unconscious are relieved. Abreaction is the process extending from catharsis to ultimate discharge of tension. Originated by JOSEF BREUER as a therapeutic technique.

Abruf (aus dem Gedächtnisreservoir) recall.
The bringing of information acquired by learning or past experience into consciousness. *Retrieval* refers more to the recovery or location of material stored in, for example, a computer (and sometimes the human) memory. → **Reproduktionsfähigkeit.**

Abstiegsneurose (VON WEIZSÄCKER) status-reduction reaction; demotion reaction.
Maladjustment brought about by a come-down in social status. *Role deprivation* could be used when individuals or groups are denied cultural and psychological status.
Examples: mandatory retirement, exclusion of minority groups from roles.

Abstinenzregel rule of abstinence; abstinence rule.
A rule imposed by the psychoanalyst that the patient should abstain from excessive sexual, aggressive, or other gratifications that might create a distraction from therapy.
cf. **Koitusverbot**.

Abstinenzsyndrom → **Entziehungserscheinungen.**

Abwehrmechanismen defense mechanisms, ego defense mechanisms, defense strategies.
Patterns of behavior or reactions intended to protect the ego from unacceptable impulses and feelings.
They are common coping mechanisms, e. g. in minimizing anxiety, but are considered pathological when they assume the form of repression or displacement. FREUD spoke of the *censorship* of the ego in this context.

Adaptationssyndrome, das allgemeine Adaptationssyndrom general adaptation syndrome (GAS).
This is SELYE's term for the total mobilization of the body's defense systems in the face of

severe stress. Some authors omit the word "general".

Ademonia → **Jammer-Depression.**

Affekt affect.
Often loosely translated as *emotion* and occasionally as *feeling tone*. In English, *affect* is a psychiatric term for experience of feeling or emotion including pain, pleasure, and ranging from the most normal to pathological emotional reactions. SIFNEOS has suggested a limitation: *Affect* is a general, personal private state of being which has both biological *and* psychological components. → **Emotion**, → **Gefühl**. *Ref.* → **Alexithymie**.

Affektausbruch cathectic discharge.
The sudden discharge of affect or psychic energy by, for example, a fit of weeping or anger.

Affektaustausch emotional response.
The term as used by RENÉ SPITZ refers particularly to the reciprocal relationship between mother and child. The alleviation of anxiety in the child during the first weeks of life by the mother's prompt response is of great importance in the infant's development.

Affektentladung cathectic discharge. → **Affektausbruch.**

affektive Knotenpunkte affective nodal points.
The term stems from MOSER and refers to the gaps in the conversation between doctor and patient, during which the patient may be summing up the doctor.

affektives Klima (RENÉ SPITZ) atmosphere of maternal care and stimulation.
This is more of a definition than a translation of the term used by SPITZ, but "affective climate" might be misunderstood unless obvious from the context. *Mothering* would be the correct in most cases, although the German refers to a situation or condition, while the English term denotes a relationship providing a child with emotional warmth and stimulation.
Ref.: Longman [7]; ALEXANDER [1].

affektive Störungen affective disorders *(DSM-III)*.
Disorders in which the affective disturbance is the primary abnormality. The present tendency is to restrict the term to conditions in which there is a protracted disturbance of mood, whether euphoric or depressive. The spectrum covered by the *DSM-III* term is shown in Fig. 1.
Ref.: PETERS [11].

Affektlahmheit affective rigidity.
Lack of emotional response to different conditions. Changing situations fail to have much effect on "feelings". Encountered mostly in schizophrenia.

Affektreaktion → **primitive Affektreaktion.**

Affektschock → **Emotionsstupor.**

Affektsperre affect block.
A condition in which fear of emotional ties prevents the patient from expressing any strong feelings. Encountered in schizophrenia and obsessive compulsion.

Affenliebe monkey love.
Doting maternal affection in which the mother tries to satisfy her child's every whim.

Agglutination → **Bildagglutination.**

Aggressionsanstauung pent-up aggression.

agieren to act out. **Agieren** acting out.
In both languages *acting out* is a psychoanalytical term denoting uncontrolled expression of impulses to gain relief. In psychotherapy it refers to release of repressed feelings, e.g. in psychodrama and children's play therapy. In uncontrolled situations it may be harmful.

The English term, *but not the German,* is sometimes applied to delinquent or antisocial behavior. In more general usage **agieren** may mean simply *to act* or gesticulate (**mit den Händen agieren** to talk with one's hands).

Aha-Erlebnis aha experience.
The pleasant reaction on gaining sudden insight into the way events or facts are connected, such as in problem solving and psychotherapy.

Akoasma acousma (plural: acousmas or acousmata); acoasm; akoasm.
An auditory hallucination of nonverbal character such as buzzing or ringing.

Aktivität → **gegenphobische Aktivität.**

Aktualisierung actualization.
Mobilizing individual potentialities and expressing them in concrete form. **Aktualisierung von Konflikten** actualization of conflicts.

akute Kampfreaktion combat reactions.
The English term comes under the DSM-III category "posttraumatic stress disorders". The more well-known term *combat fatigue* covers both physical and emotional exhaustion caused by the tensions of combat conditions. The term is synonymous with *combat exhaustion* or *operational fatigue,* but *combat hysteria* is a functional disturbance that arises so as to avoid further combat.

akute tödliche Katatonie catatonic cerebral paralysis; Stauder's lethal catatonia.
A form of schizophrenia in which an episode of motor unrest and delirium is followed by death. The origin is obscure and the condition is now rare.

Alexithymie alexithymia.
Limited fantasy and emotional life.
Ref.: SIFNEOS, P. E. et al.: The Phenomenon of Alexithymia. Proc. 11th Eur. Conf. Psychosom. Res., Heidelberg 1976, in: Psychother. Psychosom. 28 (1977) 47–57.

Algolagnie algolagnia.
Sexual feeling associated with inflicting or experiencing pain.

Alkoholdepravation → **alkoholische Wesensänderung.**

Alkoholentziehungskur detoxification.
cf. **Trinkerheilanstalt.**

Alkoholentzugssyndrom alcoholic withdrawal.
Physical and emotional symptoms arising after stopping or reducing habitual and heavy consumption of alcohol. Among the many symptoms present may be coarse tremors but not delirium tremens (which would be *alcohol-withdrawal delirium*).

alkoholischer Dämmerzustand → **pathologischer Rausch.**

alkoholischer Eifersuchtswahn alcoholic jealousy.
A particular form of alcoholic psychosis. It may remit after detoxification. The symptoms often take the form of delusional jealousy (→ **Eifersuchtswahn**). It is not classified separately in *DSM-III* but referred to as *alcohol dependence with an additional diagnosis of paranoid disorder.*

alkoholische Wesensänderung
A mild form of dementia associated with alcohol. The German term is synonymous with **Alkoholdepravation** and refers to a change in personality profile, particularly with respect to moral issues.

Allmacht der Gedanken omnipotence of thought.
FREUD's expression for the feeling or fear that wishes can become reality. First observed in compulsive neurosis, the thought is reflected

in normally healthy people by sending greetings and good wishes on festive occasions.

Alphatraining alpha-wave training.
A form of biofeedback in which an individual is trained to achieve a relaxed state by control of his alpha waves, usually by the aid of a signal tone which changes when the alpha state is reached.

Alter age. → **Rückbildungsalter.**

Altersdepression depression of late onset; involutional depression.
Endogenous depression occurring in or after middle age. The patients have had no prior symptoms. → **Rückbildungsalter.**

alternierendes Bewusstsein, alternierende Persönlichkeit alternating personality (SOLBRIG).
A type of personality that causes an individual to lead a double life. *Example:* A devoted housewife who, at certain intervals, say, after a sleep, works as a prostitute. → **Persönlichkeitsspaltung.**

Altersschwachsinn dotage = feebleness of mind in old age; senility.
In severe and more specific cases this may be one of the senile psychoses resulting from degeneration of the brain in old age.

Altgedächtnis remote memory.
Retrieval of events or information from the distant past. Characteristic of many of the elderly.

Ambitendenz ambitendency.
The presence of opposing behavioral drives. However, when **Ambivalenz des Wollens** in BLEULER's sense is meant, *ambivalence of the will* would be preferable. This is observed in schizophrenia, when the patient may, for example, desire to eat and not to eat.

Ammenschlaf-Phänomen sleep vigil.
Sleep undisturbed by habitual sounds but broken by significant noise. *Example:* A mother or nurse may sleep through a thunderstorm or traffic noise but awake on hearing a child cry.

Amnesie → **transitorische globale Amnesie.**

anaklitische Depression *Syn.:* **Anlehnungsdepression** anaclitic depression.
A form of depression in infants separated from their mothers. It is characterized by an expressionless face, despondency and lethargy. The condition is reversible on resumption of mothering care.

Analphabetismus illiteracy → **emotionaler Analphabetismus.**

Analyse analysis → **bioenergetische Analyse,** → **gezielte Analyse,** → **Kontrollanalyse,** → **Kurzanalyse,** → **Lehranalyse,** → **Schicksalsanalyse,** → **Transaktionsanalyse.**

analytische Psychologie analytic (or analytical) psychology.
The term refers to the hypotheses of C. G. JUNG. It also covers those disciplines that use free association, hypnosis, abreaction, and narcoanalysis in order to uncover defense mechanisms leading to conflict and neurosis.

Anamnese case history. → **Fremdanamnese.**

anerkennende Haltung commendatory attitude.

Anfall attack; fit; seizure; bout; access.
All the English terms refer to the sudden onset of a disease or its symptoms, and the distinctions made in common usage can be learned only by examples, a few of which are listed: an attack of bronchitis, an asthmatic attack; an epileptic fit (or seizure), a bout of shivering, a fit of rage; an akinetic seizure (or any other condition associated with convul-

sions); a bout (or paroxysm) of coughing, a bout of fever, a severe bout of backache; an access of paralysis (rarer).
→ **psychomotorischer Anfall,** → **Tobsuchtsanfall,** → **Unzinatusanfall,** → **Wachanfall.**

Anfälligkeit proneness, susceptibility.
→ **Unfallanfälligkeit.**

angeborene Auslösemechanismen (AAM) innate releasing mechanisms; inherited releasing mechanisms (IRM).
Behavioral patterns in animals that are inborn rather than conditioned by stimulus, but are triggered by specific environmental factors or signals.

angepasst adapted.
angepasste Patienten adapted patients. This is the second group of DEGRECOUSTRY's classification of infarct patients. Adopted by PETZOLD for determining the type of psychotherapy indicated.

Angreifer → **Identifizierung mit dem Angreifer.**

Angst anxiety.
In psychoanalysis a vague feeling of dread or of being threatened with no clear, or even conscious external cause. The feeling is often disproportionate to the danger involved. Anxiety is a signal of internal danger, stemming in many cases from unconscious conflicts. → **Furcht** (fear). From the two definitions given in this book (a synthesis of German and English definitions) it may appear that **Angst** = *anxiety,* and **Furcht** = *fear,* but in practice there is a unidirectional overlap: **Angst** may sometimes be translated by fear but **Furcht** rarely by anxiety. This is illustrated by the following *examples:* **Existenzangst** existential anxiety; **krankhafte Angst vor dem Versagen** morbid fear of failure (kakorrhaphiophobia – though WEBSTER appears to favor *dread* in the case of phobia); **Todesangst** = **Todesfurcht** fear of death.
cf. also → **Bettangst,** → **freiflottierende Angst,** → **Gewissensangst,** → **Kastrationsangst,** → **Lebensangst,** → **Nachtangst,** → **neurotische Angst,** → **psychotische Angst,** → **Realangst,** → **Vitalangst.**

Angst-Glücks-Psychose anxiety elation psychosis.
The term stems from LEONHARD (1957) and refers to one of the cycloid psychoses. The condition is bipolar and is marked by changes in mood: hallucinations and delusions of reference at one pole and elation or ecstasy at the other.
Ref.: Oxford Textbook of Psychiatry [6], p. 243.

Angstdämpfung relief of anxiety; control of anxiety.

Angstdepression anxiety depression; anxious depression.
A form of depression (mostly endogenous) in which anxiety predominates but agitation is lacking.

Angsthierarchie anxiety hierarchy.
The listing of a patient's fears, or stimuli producing them, in order of intensity. These range from minor stimuli producing anxiety ("Did I lock the door before leaving?") at the bottom of the list to major stimuli in the form of, say, very disturbing news, death of a near relative, etc., at the top. Desensitization, of a phobia for example, is then begun with the least threatening situation, after which the others are tackled in turn. Important techniques employed in this method of treatment are autogenic training or JACOBSON's relaxation exercises.

Angstschweiß cold sweat.

Angstverarbeitung coping with anxiety.
cf. → **Verarbeitung**

Anklage accusation. → **Selbstanklage.**

Anlehnenwollen need for dependence.
The desire to have someone to lean on; anaclitic need.

Anlehnungsdepression → **anaklitische Depression.**

Anlehnungstendenzen tendencies towards dependency; (stronger) anaclitic tendencies.
The child has an *anaclitic* relation to its mother: it *leans on* her for everything.

Anpassung adjustment.
In psychiatry the term refers to the process of modifying one's emotional life and behavior in order to conform to social norms and deal with a variety of difficult situations.

Anpassungsstörungen adjustment disorder *(DSM-III),* adjustment reaction *(ICD-9);* adaptation reaction.
There are several categories: adjustment disorder (a.d.) with depressed mood; a.d. with anxious mood; a.d. with mixed emotional features; a.d. with disturbance of conduct; a.d. with mixed disturbance of emotions and conduct; a.d. with work or academic inhibition; a.d. with withdrawal; a.d. with atypical features. Such maladaptive disorders are usually situation-specific and generally reversible. They occur shortly after a stressful situation such as divorce, separation, retirement, or occupational problems.

Anspruchsniveau aspiration level; level of aspiration.
The standards of performance an individual sets for himself.

Ansteckung → **Gefühlsansteckung.**

Antikonvulsiva antiepileptics.
Drugs used to lower the frequency of epileptic attacks or to treat them once they are in progress.

Antrieb drive; initiative.
Organized effort to achieve a special purpose. This is a different sense of "drive" than that sometimes employed for → **Trieb,** being a broader concept involving the intellect, and having a rather elusive quality that is linked closely to the individual personality structure. It is pathologically increased in manic states, where it could be called *impulse* (pyromania is a disorder of impulse control) and severely decreased in depression.
Examples: **Ihm fehlt jeder Antrieb** he lacks drive. **Fehlen des Spontanantriebs** lack of initiative and willpower (as in abulia), or (more general) loss of drive. **Aus eigenem Antrieb** on one's own initiative. **Die Belohnung verlieh ihm neuen Antrieb** the reward gave him fresh incentive. Several other alternatives exist in nonpsychological contexts.
cf. → **Zwangsantrieb.**

antriebssteigende Antidepressiva; aktivierende oder hemmungslösende Antidepressiva drive-enhancing antidepressants; inhibition unblocking antidepressants.

Apathie → **emsige Apathie.**

Apparat → **psychischer Apparat.**

Apperzeption apperception.
Awareness of meaning and significance of an object. Clear perception or recognition. *Verb:* to apperceive. In historical texts the term may refer to a concept of JOHANN HERBART (1776–1841): below the conscious threshold, ideas compete for apperceptive attention until the strongest triumphs and becomes conscious.

Appetenz appetency, appetence.
An instinctive inclination to perform certain actions, usually for the gratification of desires, e.g. nutritional or sexual.

Appetenzverhalten appetitive behavior.
Usually excessive or deficient eating. Lesions

of the ventromedial nucleus cause voracious eating, those of the lateral hypothalamic nuclei result in anorexia.

Arbeit → **Trauerarbeit,** → **Traumarbeit.**

Arzneimittelmißbrauch drug abuse.
The use of drugs without therapeutic indication. *Drug misuse* refers to the incorrect use of medically indicated drugs. *Substance abuse (DSM-III)* includes alcohol and infers resultant impairment of social behavior and inability to cut down on intake. On this latter point the term agrees with the German in that the condition borders on addiction (→ **Sucht**).
Ref.: H. Coper: What is drug dependence? (editorial) Pharmacopsychiat. 18 (1985) 323–324; Longman Dictionary [7].

Assekurose compensation neurosis; indemnity neurosis.
The tendency to exaggerate the importance of disability or illness in order to gain high insurance compensation.

Assoziation → **Erinnerungsassoziation,** → **freie Assoziation,** → **Klangassoziation.**

asthmatisches Keuchen asthmatic wheeze.

Asymbolie → **Schmerzasymbolie.**

A-Typ (Persönlichkeitsbild) Type A (personality).
A person having a life-style predisposing to coronary heart disease: highly competitive, fatigue suppressed, hostile when frustrated (after Friedman and Rosenman, U.S.A). Richter and Beckmann (Germany) see this person as having a "clinging" nature and being a victim of his dependence. *cf.* → **B-Typ.**

atypische stereotype Bewegungsstörung atypical stereotyped-movement disorder (DSM-III).
Unlike the tics included under stereotyped-movement disorders (→ **stereotype Bewegungsstörungen**), the movements in this disorder are voluntary and do not appear to cause distress, even though they may consist of head-banging, rocking, and other rhythmic movements. The disorder is encountered in childhood.

audiogene Krämpfe audiogenic seizure.
An epileptiform seizure brought on by sound waves.

aufdeckende Psychotherapie depth therapy; uncovering techniques.
Psychotherapeutic techniques in which repressed material and conflicts are brought to the surface of the consciousness. Hence, psychoanalysis is invariably an uncovering technique, no matter what form it adopts.
cf. **zudeckende Psychotherapie.**

Auffassung
In cases where the German expression means **Aufnahme von Wahrnehmungs- und Vorstellungsmaterial** (Peters [11]) the nearest English equivalent would appear to be *grasp,* particularly as Webster defines this as a "mental hold or comprehension" and *to grasp* as "to lay hold on with the mind". Unfortunately this is not a current psychological term like **Auffassung,** which also involves the principle of **Prägnanz** (→ **Prägnanzregel),** and the most common translations are *comprehension* and *perception.* In some cases, depending on the context, *perceptivity* would be more appropriate, though this is more **Auffassungsvermögen.**

Auffassungsstörung a lack or weakness of mental grasp.
Perceptual deficit could be used when referring to a case of impaired ability to interpret sensory experience in a meaningful manner, grasp a situation or understand people and concepts.

Aufforderungscharakter valence.
The quality attributed by Lewin to certain symbols, objects and constellations in affect-

ing behavior. Those repelling an individual (or organism) are said to have negative valence, while those attracting have positive valence. The expression stems from LEWIN's "field theory" (→ **Feldtheorie des Verhaltens).**

aufgeben to give up, to surrender. → **Selbstaufgabe.**

Aufklärung, sexuelle → sexuelle Aufklärung.

Aufmerksamkeitsdefizit → Störung mit Aufmerksamkeitsdefizit.

Aufnahme admission (to a hospital); uptake (absorption and incorporation of a substance by living tissue).

Aufschlussdiagnose = Differentialdiagnose differential diagnosis.

Ausbreitung → Gedankenausbreitung.

Ausbruch → Affektausbruch.

Ausdruckshader expressive slips.
Accidents and errors in speech that "betray" neurotic patients.

Ausdruckskrankheiten conversion disorders; hysterical neuroses, conversion type (according to context).
cf. **Konversion. Ausdruckskrankheit** was the expression employed VON UEXKÜLL, who used it as distinct from → **Bereitstellungskrankheiten**. He considered the symptoms of conversion disorders to have **Ausdrucksbedeutung** (expressive significance).

Ausdrucksphänomene → minimale Ausdrucksphänomene.

ausflippen to flip out; to freak out.
The German expression would appear to be derived from the American English *to flip out* which, however, means to lose self-control. *To freak out* is somewhat stronger, meaning to withdraw from reality and society, particularly by taking drugs, and behave in an irrational, unconventional manner. It also implies nightmarish hallucinations after a "bad trip".
Ref.: WEBSTER's Third New International Dictionary, Addenda.

ausgebrannt burned-out.
An expression describing primarily schizophrenic patients, or rather those suffering from process psychosis, who have become withdrawn, apathetic and anergic. Such espressions as *burned-out schizophrenic* or *anergic schizophrenic* are also used.
cf. **Prozeßschizophrenie.**

Ausgleichen to compensate.
Eine Kränkung ausgleichen to compensate a mortification, offense or injury.

Auslösemechanismen release mechanisms.
→ **angeborene Auslösemechanismen.**

aussersinnliche Wahrnehmung extrasensory perception (ESP); paranormal cognition.
A collective term for awareness of events obtained by means other than those involving normal sensory channels. These include telepathy, clairvoyance and precognition, all of which belong to the controversial realm of parapsychology.

ausstossen to exclude, to reject, to expel.
→ **Stadium des Ausstossens.**

Austausch exchange. → **Affektaustausch.**

Austragungsweisen conversion,
E.g. **leibliche Austragungsweisen** physical conversion. An unusual construction; the German expression generally employed is → **Konversion** or **Konversionssymptome.** *N. B.* **Austragen** has a host of other meanings: to deliver, settle, contest, carry a baby to full term.

Automatie → **Befehlsautomatie.**

Automismusverlust (L. SÜLLWOLD) loss of common skills or abilities (combing the hair, shaving, etc.).
If this is marked by absence of energy or extreme passivity the term *anergia* could be employed, and *stupor* when the individual is unresponsive and immobile.

Automorphismus automorphic perception.
The tendency to perceive and judge others in accordance with one's own criteria without considering the differences.

Autophagie autophagia.
The desire to eat, or actual eating of, one's own flesh.

archaisches Denken archaic thought.
This is similar to *concrete thinking* (→ **konkretes Denken**), but that the thought processes lack any form of reasoning. Concreteness, immediate perception, and feeling dominate to such an extent that no thought is accorded to objective differences: everything is self-evident.

Aversions-Aversions-Konflikt avoidance-avoidance conflict; double avoidance conflict.
The choice between two equally threatening or objectionable situations.

B

Bambergersche Krankheit saltatory spasm; Bamberger's disease; saltatory tic.
Clonic muscle spasm of the legs producing jumping or dancing movements as soon as the soles of the feet touch the ground.

Bambinos *(Drogenjargon)* bennies; (singular: benny).
The English slang equivalent is derived from *Benzedrine*®. A tablet, usually of amphetamine, taken as a stimulant.

barbituratfreie Beruhigungsmittel non-barbiturate sedatives.

Basisneuroleptika "basic neuroleptics".
The term was originally introduced by GROSS and KALTENBÄCK in 1967 to cover the broad-spectrum neuroleptics having a marked sedative and hypnogenic effect.
→ **Neuroleptika.**

Beachtungswahn delusion of observation. *cf.* **Beziehungswahn.**

bedingter Reflex conditioned reflex.
Acquired or learned response to a stimulus that did not formerly elicit response before conditioning. Also called *conditioned response.*

Bedrückung dejection.

Bedürfnis need. → **physiologisches Bedürfnis, primäres Bedürfnis,** → **sekundäres Bedürfnis,** → **reaktives Bedürfnis.**

Beeinflussung → **Gedankenbeeinflussung,** → **leibliches Beeinflussungserlebnis.**

Beeinflussungsgefühl delusion of influence.
A disturbance in ego functions under which the patient falsely believes he is being subjected to external influence or control, e.g. from hypnosis or radio waves. Typical of schizophrenia.

Befehlsautomatie automatic obedience.
The slavish, mechanical, and unhesitant copying or repetition of the speech and actions of others. Most frequently encountered in catatonic schizophrenia.

Befriedigung → **Ersatzbefriedigung.**

Befund → **psychischer Befund.**

Befürchtungen → **Zwangsbefürchtungen.**

Begehrensneurose = **Begehrungsneurose** → **Assekurose.**

Begleiterscheinungen concomitant effects.
A term preferred by some authors to **Nebenwirkungen** (side effects) when speaking of psychopharmaceuticals.

Begleitstimmen auditory hallucination; hearing of voices.
According to K. SCHNEIDER this constitutes one of the most definite symptoms in diagnosing schizophrenia, but the phenomenon can also occur in other psychoses and in alcoholism.

Beglückungserlebnis elation.
A feeling of intense joy that may be ecstatic and restless. It is an important symptom in manic states, but may occur in other mental disorders. Unless it is clear from the context that "elation" is a psychiatric symptom, it would be better to precede the English term by the adjective *exaggerated*, since in everyday language it may just mean "high spirits".

Begnadigungswahn delusion of pardon.
A facet of prison psychosis in which a prisoner serving a long sentence becomes convinced that he will be pardoned.

Behandlung → **Schlafentzugsbehandlung.**

Behandlungsmassnahmen → **Nichtbefolgen der ärztlichen Behandlungsmassnahmen.**

"Be-Haupt-ung"
This is an example of a German play on words used in psychosomatics, in this case to describe an emotional condition in cervicalgia: **emotional erschwerte Be-Haupt-ung.** The nearest translation (leaving aside the pun) would be *emotionally impeded self-maximation.* The latter term refers to the drive to maintain feelings of adequacy through competitive situations.

Behinderung handicap. → **geistige Behinderung.**

Behütung → **übermässige Behütung**

Beichtskrupel scrupels of confession; scrupulosity.
The German term refers to the fear observed in compulsive patients that they might have omitted details in confessing something and will find no peace of mind until the confession is complete. The first English term is rather literal and the second more comprehensive, meaning that the patient attaches great importance to details and is overconcerned with what is right or wrong.

Belastung burden; strain; stress.
These English equivalents are restricted to the psychological field. *Burden* is a rather general term which could also denote a chronic affliction as well as a particularly difficult duty. There is a great overlap between *strain* and *stress.* The latter appears rather fashionable nowadays when speaking of illness, whereas anyone may be under strain at some time without it having any psychiatric or psychosomatic significance. Such persons are not necessarily suffering from stress, yet it is difficult to envisage any person under strain who is not stressed.

Benehmen → **läppisches Benehmen.**

Benommenheit a benumbed state; drowsiness.
The first term is more of a definition that may be used in a general sense. The German term is, however, often synonymous with **Somnolenz,** which could mean *sleepiness* or *drowsiness,* the pathological term being *somnolence,* the first degree of clouding of consciousness (→ **Bewusstseinstrübung**). When used in BLEULER's original sense referring to acute schizophrenic disturbances involving slowed mental processes, the original German expression is sometimes retained in English.

Beobachtung observation → **Selbstbeobachtung.**

Beratung → **Erziehungsberatungsstellen,** → **Kinderberatung.**

Bereitschaft → **Komplexbereitschaft.**

Beruhigungsmittel sedative(s) → **barbituratfreie Beruhigungsmittel.**

Benzinismus gasoline sniffing (U.S.); petrol sniffing (U.K.)
The more official term is *gasoline intoxication,* which refers to the euphoric feeling induced by inhaling gasoline vapor, and comes under the main heading of *volatile-chemical inhalation.*

Bereitstellungskrankheiten disorders of the disposition of emotions which anticipate or prepare one for action (WEINER).
This may be shortened to *disorders of the disposition of emotions.* A further suggestion is *disturbances in states of preparedness.* The original German term stems from VON UEX-

KÜLL, whose work on psychosomatic disorders has not been translated into English. **Bereitstellungskrankheiten** have also been termed *so-called psychosomatic disorders,* sometimes classified under somatoform disorders, and at others considered a special case of conversion symptoms (→ **Ausdruckskrankheiten**). The important thing to remember is that no action occurs but physiological and structural changes take place. Emotions are undischarged so one could also speak of *disorders of undischarged emotion.*

Ref.: Psychiatry: Medical Outline Series [5], p. 184.

Berufsneurose → **Beschäftigungsneurose.**

Berufungswahn messianic delusion.
The false conviction of being called upon by higher or divine powers to improve the lot of mankind. The English term given is rare but corresponds more closely to the German than the more frequently used term *delusions of grandeur,* which has wider implications.
cf. **Grössenwahn.**

Beschäftigungsneurose occupational neurosis.
A reaction to anxiety and tension that impairs or prevents the patient carrying out his work. A well-known example is writer's cramp.

beschützende Werkstätte sheltered workshop.
A workshop for the resocialization of discharged patients who are still incapable of being fully reintegrated into the normal work scene. They are given useful employment and receive pay, but the workshop is run on a non-profitmaking basis.

Besessenheit demonic possession; demoniac possession; obsession; frenzy; madness.
The German term goes back to a widespread belief held up to the nineteenth century that illness could be attributed to evil spirits gaining possession of the body or of the soul. In more liberal usage it will be found to be equivalent to *obsession.* **Von etwas besessen sein:** to be obsessed with something. Technically speaking, "obsession" ranges from benign intrusions on the consciousness to obsessive fears and images from traumatic events.

Besetzung cathexis.
Investment of psychic energy or drive in any "object", which may be a person or a group of people, an idea, the self, or a fantasy. *Adjective:* cathected.
→ **Gegenbesetzung,** → **Libidobesetzung.**

Besinnung consciousness.
Examples: **bei Besinnung sein** to be conscious; **wieder zur Besinnung kommen** to regain consciousness. However, the word has other connotations depending on the context. In the sense employed by E. STÖRRING the term means more than *recollection* and even *retrospection* and extends to *an evaluation of the past.*

Betäubungsmittelsucht narcomania; narcotic addiction.
The first term refers to a pathological desire for narcotics, whereas the second is stronger, meaning that addiction is present and there is a tendency to increase the dose with mounting tolerance.

Betäubungstrinker escape drinker.
Excessive alcohol intake in order to relieve pain or escape from tension. This comes under the heading of *alpha alcoholism.*

Bettangst bed phobia.
The fear of going to bed, possibly because of initial insomnia (→ **Einschlafstörungen**).

Bettsucht bed craving.
A pathologically increased need for sleep and spending long periods in bed even without sleep. It often constitutes a flight from the difficulties of daily existence into the warm shelter of the bed. May be a symptom of endogenous depression.

Bewegungsdrang hyperactivity; hyperkinesia; hyperkinesis.
Persistent unrest and overactivity, particularly in manic states and in brain-damaged or emotionally disturbed children.

Bewegungssperre akinesia.
Absence of muscle tone and control of voluntary movement, e.g. in catatonic states.

Bewegungsstereotypie stereotypy.
Automatic and persistent repetition of movements or words. It is common in catatonic schizophrenia and autism.
→ **stereotype Bewegungsstörungen.**

Bewegungsstörungen movement disorders.
→ **stereotype Bewegungsstörungen,** → **atypische stereotype Bewegungsstörung,** → **stereotype Bewegungsstörungen.**

Bewusstlosigkeit unconsciousness.
In its extreme form *coma* (→ **Koma).**

Bewusstsein consciousness.
The state and content of the mind in response to impressions made by the senses: a current state of awareness. In English, *the conscious* refers to a part of the mind or a level of consciousness in the psychoanalytic sense. **Bewusstseinseinengung** narrowing of the field of consciousness. **bewusstseinsfern** (adj.) well below the conscious level.
The above are psychoanalytical interpretations; the psychopathological levels are given under → **klares Bewusstsein,** → **Benommenheit,** → **Bewusstlosigkeit.**
cf. also → **Ichbewusstsein,** → **Leibbewusstsein,** → **Randbewusstsein,** → **Spaltung des Bewusstseins.**

Bewusstseinstrübung clouding of consciousness; mental fog.
A quantitative impairment of consciousness which makes it difficult to get through to the patient. It is often a sign of acute organic brain damage, infections or toxic disorders. For the various degrees of intensity → **Benommenheit,** → **Sopor,** → **Koma.**

Beziehungsfalle double bind.
Usually a familial situation in which the child receives contradictory messages from one or both parents. The mother may, for example, complain of the child's lack of affection yet reject any outward manifestation of it.

Beziehungsstörung attachment disorder.
Failure of infants to thrive owing to isolation or emotional neglect. **Reaktive Beziehungsstörung (im Säuglingsalter)** reactive-attachment disorder of infancy. This is also a DSM-III term and refers to a lack of normal responsiveness in a child owing to the absence of care and affection. The young patient fails to smile, is apathetic, and ocular pursuit is lacking.

Beziehungstherapie relationship therapy.
Psychotherapy in which the relationship between patient and therapist is a key factor.

Beziehungswahn delusion of reference.
The pathological interpretation of a patient who believes that everything being said or written in his environment refers to himself. He may also have the feeling of being watched.

Bezugsperson person of reference.
A person to whom an individual has a particularly strong bond of feeling, projection playing a major role.

Bildagglutination image agglutination(s).
The merging of several different shapes or pictures into a whole, e.g. in dreams. In the wider sense the term may refer to the condensing of several concepts into a single picture.

Bilderleben → **katathymes Bilderleben.**

Bildstreifendenken hypnagogic imagery.
A series of pictures occurring during a super-

ficial dream state just before falling to sleep or during drowsiness.

Bildung formation; education. → **Reaktionsbildung.**

Bindungslosigkeit lack of (affiliative) bonding.
The absence of any emotional attachment or interpersonal relationships, as may occur in drug addicts or sociopathic personalities.

bioenergetische Analyse bioenergetics.
The theory behind this form of psychotherapy is that the human organism accumulates and discharges energy; should this system be disturbed, muscular tension and illness result. The treatment has been defined as follows: "A way of relieving the individual's chronic muscular tensions and rigidities resulting from emotional stress and unresolved emotional conflicts." A. LOWEN's approach involves movement, respiration, and posture therapy. It is based on the work of W. REICH.

biologisches Gedächtnis
1. genetic memory.
Information based on learning may be stored in a DNA or RNA molecule and thus inherited as part of a chromosome.
2. genetic storage.
Information based on learning stored by the nervous system at synaptic or metabolic levels. It has been suggested that this not only forms a basis for instinctual behavior in animals but also for the collective unconscious.

Blickkontakt eye contact.
The reciprocal act of two individuals looking each other in the eyes, usually in order to enhance communication. *Example:* Eye contact between mother and child plays an important role in emotional development.

Blindheit → **funktionelle Blindheit,** → **hysterische Blindheit,** → **psychogene Blindheit.**

Blitz-Nick-Salaam-Krämpfe (BNS-Krämpfe) nodding spasm, salaam spasm, salaam convulsions.
Clonic spasm of the sternomastoid muscles producing bowing movements. → **Krampf.**

Bovarismus bovarism.
Inability to distinguish between reality and dream content or fantasy (after the heroine of Gustave Flaubert's book, *Madame Bovary).*

Boxerenzephalopathie = Boxerdemenz Boxer's dementia.
A chronic disorder of the brain resulting from repeated head punches. Commonly known as *punch-drunkenness* or *being punch-drunk.* In English, *boxer's dementia* is the more advanced form, while *boxer's traumatic encephalopathy* is the more general term.

Breitbandneuroleptika broad-spectrum neuroleptics (by analogy with the broad-spectrum antibiotics).
A group of psychopharmaceuticals particularly suited to treating acute anxiety, severe agitation, emotional tension, or a combination of such symptoms. Examples are promazine and chlorprothixene. → **Langzeitneuroleptika,** → Figure 3.
Ref.: W. PÖLDINGER: Compendium of Psychopharmacotherapy, p. 119. Editiones Roche, Basle 1984.

Breuer-Verfahren cathartic method.
A method introduced by JOSEF BREUER in which the patient was induced to talk about sexual feelings while under hypnosis.

B-Typ (Persönlichkeitsbild) 1. Type B (personality).
A personality pattern that enables an individual to relax without feeling guilty, or work without needing to prove himself (after FRIEDMAN and ROSENMANN, USA). RICHTER and BECKMANN (Germany) see this person as one attempting to keep down the helpless feeling of dependence by banning it from his

consciousness and containing it by a show of energy or overactivity. → **A-Typ.**

2. B-Typ (nach Jaensch) B type.
This refers to a type of eidetic imagery that is both transient and changeable, being evoked by pure imagination. → **T-Typ.**

Bulimarexie bulmorexia.
A disorder in which episodes of voracious eating *(binges)* are followed by self-induced vomiting. The condition is sometimes described as the *purging-gorging syndrome.*

C

Capgras-Zeichen Capgras' syndrome.
The meaning becomes clear on translating the original French term *L'illusion des sosies* (the illusion of doubles). However, this is not really an illusion, but more of a delusional misinterpretation (→ **Sinnestäuschung,** → **Wahn**). The patient has difficulty in identifying persons known to him and *believes* they are merely doubles, insisting on supposed or imaginary differences in their appearance. This should not be confused with the mania described by SERIEUX and CAPGRAS known as "folie raisonnante" (→ **Räsoniermanie**).
Ref.: Oxford Textbook of Psychiatry [6], p. 5.

Charakter → **oraler Charakter,** → **syntoner Charakter.**

Charaktereigentümlichkeiten traits (of character).

Charakterpanzerung character armor.
A pattern of reaction firmly anchored in an individual's personality to serve as a defense against anxiety or penetration into the unconscious. The reaction may take the form of aggressiveness, cynicism, and attempts to conceal facial expressions and other personal manifestations. The term was first used in the analytic sense by WILHELM REICH.

chronische motorische Ticstörung chronic motor-tic disorder (DSM-III).
Involuntary twitches involving up to three muscle groups. The disorder persists for a year or more.

Cocktailparty-Syndrom chatterbox effect; cocktail-party conversationalism.
One of the behavioral facets of hydrocephalus patients. Superficially the patient appears quite capable of social conversation, but on closer analysis he is found to be incapable of meaningful communication.

D

Dämmerattacke → **psychomotorischer Anfall.**

Dämmerschlaf twilight sleep.
A sleepy state in which awareness is dulled and the memory of any pain is effaced. It may occur naturally or be prolonged for therapeutic purposes by hypnotics. For childbirth it is sometimes induced by a barbiturate and scopolamine.

Dämmerzustand twilight state.
In everyday language the German expression originally referred to inattention and absentmindedness. These impressions are still part of the picture but the psychiatric term implies additional signs and symptoms. Briefly, it is generally agreed to be a clouding of the consciousness, unawareness of surroundings, transient hallucinations, memory gaps afterwards and acts out of keeping with the patient's normal pattern of behavior. The condition may occur in epilepsy, brain damage, or under the influence of drugs.
→ **alkoholischer Dämmerzustand.**

dämpfen to depress, inhibit, damp down.
Generally, one depresses a system and inhibits a function. Emotions can be *damped down,* and **Dämpfung der Erregbarkeit** may in many cases be rendered by *control of agitation.*

dargebotene Hand, Die → **Telefonseelsorge.**

Darreichungsform dosage form (of a pharmaceutical product).

Daseinsanalyse Dasein analysis.
Strictly speaking this term refers to the philosophic/phenomological approach for not only realizing *'where we are'* but what we can become, the aim being to help people help themselves.
Existential analysis refers to a phase in existential psychotherapy in which a person is encouraged to examine his own sense of values and commitments and achieve greater fulfillment. One speaks of *dasein analysis* when referring to the psychotherapeutic procedure initiated by BINSWANGER, which is derived from the philosophical approach of HEIDEGGER or HUSSERL, while one speaks of *existential analysis* when the principles of logotherapy are involved – which employ existential philosophy as their point of departure. In current practice this term is often used to translate **Daseinsanalyse** since there is considerable overlap.

Dauerschlaf 1. prolonged sleep.
Sleep extending long over normal periods, over days or even weeks.
2. A synonym for **Schlafkur:** sleep treatment or prolonged narcosis. Rarely used today.

Daumenlutschen thumb-sucking.
Wonnesaugen (literally "pleasure sucking") is a rare term.

"Dazwischen-Sein" falling between two stools.
SEEMANN's description of a condition in patients bound up with their symptoms who show marked resistance to any form of psychotherapy. Their symptoms are painful but of a functional nature. Uncertainty and lability lead such patients to seek out a doctor who will confirm the presence of a physical complaint.

Debilität mild mental retardation.
The IQ suggested for the mildest form of mental retardation is 70–80. The German

term should not be confused with the English word *debility*, which refers more to physical weakness or infirmity.

Deckerinnerung screen memory, cover memory.
Memory of slightly unpleasant or shameful experiences in early childhood, the purpose of which is to cover up such a memory of greater significance. This form of resistance is encountered in psychoanalysis.

Defektsyndrom → terminales extrapyramidales Defektsyndrom.

Delegation delegation.
The tendency of some parents to ignore their children's true abilities and press them into fulfilling their own unachieved ambitions.

Delir → Fieberdelir, → mussitierendes Delirium.

Denken thinking, thought, imagery.
→ archaisches Denken, → Bildstreifendenken, → Einschlafdenken, → inhaltliche Denkstörungen, → operatives Denken, → sprunghaftes Denken, → synkretes Denken.

Denksperre blocking, mental block; thought obstruction; thought deprivation.
Sudden, involuntary interruptions in the flow of speech or thought, which may be restored after a certain period. In schizophrenia the block may be prolonged, while it can also occur for short periods in normal persons affected by disturbing events.

Denkstörung thought disorder. **→ inhaltliche Denkstörung.**

Denktypus → extravertierter Denktypus, → introvertierter Denktypus.

Depersonalisation → Wirklichkeitsentfremdung.

Depravation depravation; a change for the worse. **→ Alkoholdepravation.**

Depression depression. **→ Altersdepression, → anaklitische Depression, → Angstdepression, → Anlehnungsdepression, → Erschöpfungsdepression, → involutive Depression, → Jammer-Depression, → klagsam-agitierte Depression, → larvierte Depression, → maskierte Depression, → weinerlich-agitierte Depression.**

Depressions-Schmerz-Syndrom depression-pain syndrome.
Recently adopted in the USA, the term covers all common states of depression accompanied by pain except in cases where the pain must be considered a clearly separate disease on the basis of its etiology. This comes under the main heading of *masked depression* (**→ larvierte Depression**).
Ref.: HARENKO, A.: Low back pain in connection with depression. Hexagon 'Roche' 13, No. 2 (1985) 9–12. Also in German: idem, Kreuzschmerz und Depression.

Depressivität depressive moods.

Derealisation → Wirklichkeitsentfremdung.

Dermatitis autogenica dermatitis artefacta.
Self-inflicted skin lesions, e.g. by heat or chemicals.

Dermatozoenwahn dermatozoic delusion.
The conviction that some form of minute animal life has invaded the skin. Continual washing may produce scaling or other side effects, which confirm the patient's impression. *Formication* refers to the hallucinatory sensation of this and *acarophobia* to the fear.

desynchronisierter oder dissoziierter Schlaf → paradoxer Schlaf.

Diagnose → Gesamtdiagnose, → Aufschlussdiagnose

Differentialdiagnose → **Aufschlussdiagnose.**

direktiv-suggestive Gruppenpsychotherapie directive group psychotherapy.
A type of therapy designed by S. R. Slavson to help participants to adjust better to their environment. It includes counseling, didactic approaches, and recreation.

Dirnenphantasien prostitution fancies.
A form a daydreaming in which some women entertain the idea of being a prostitute. Euphemisms would in some cases be *hetaeral fantasy* or *courtesan fantasy,* in which a woman plays the imaginary role of a courtesan or a man plays with the idea of possessing one.

Doppelbindung → **Beziehungsfalle.**

Doppeldenken audible thought.
The patient "hears" his own thoughts and concludes that others can hear them. He has, moreover, the impression that the thoughts spring from some inner voice. This is not a true hallucination, but due to false conceptions and thus more of a delusion. → **Gedankenlautwerden**.

Doppelgängererlebnis Doppelgänger phenomenon.
The false conviction of having a double who acts and thinks the same as oneself. When this is frequently repeated it may be described in German as **Doppelgängerwahn.** For the clinical implications → **Heautoskopie.**

doppeltes Bewusstsein → **Persönlichkeitsspaltung.**

Drang impulse, craving; urge; distress.
→ **Bewegungsdrang,** → **Lebensdrang.**

Dranghandlung impulsive behavior.
Usually, sudden acts undertaken without preliminary deliberation and without considering the consequences. Such acts may be of a criminal nature and carried out under the influence of a compelling urge. *Irresistible impulse* is a forensic term; if successfully pleaded, it exempts the criminal under Common Law. *cf.* **Kurzschlußhandlung.**

Drehtürpsychiatrie revolving-door phenomenon.
Repeated readmission of patients to hospital owing to discharge before adequate diagnosis, treatment, or recovery.

"Droge Arzt" drug "doctor".
An expression coined by M. Balint suggesting that the personality and behavior of the doctor can work as a drug. Another way of writing the term is *the drug, doctor.*
Ref.: Brett, E. M.: Children with headaches. Brit. med. J. 291 (1985) 340.

Durcharbeiten working through.
An essential process in psychoanalysis in which the patient integrates interpretations, gradually overcomes resistance to the disclosure of repressed material, accepts it, and thus gains insight.

Durchschlafstörungen intermittent insomnia.
Periods of sleeplessness occurring several times nightly followed by difficulty in falling to sleep again.

dyskinetische Spätsyndrome (plur.) tardive dyskinesia.
A condition induced particularly in elderly patients or those with brain damage by prolonged administration of neuroleptics. The symptoms consist of repetitive movements such as facial grimaces, rolling of the tongue, rotation of the chin and twisting of the head to one side. Such symptoms persist even after withdrawal of the drug and may resist specific treatment.
Syn.: **Spätdyskinesien** (plur.) is the term preferred by Matussek and Hippius; → **terminales extrapyramidales Defektsyndrom.**

E

Ehefähigkeit; Ehemündigkeit marriageability; nubility.
The German terms refers to the right to enter into the state of matrimony. Particularly when one speaks of an **Ehefähigkeitszeugnis** there is no true English equivalent, although American consulates issue a "marriage affidavit", while British consulates in Switzerland will provide a "certificate of law".

Ehepaartherapie conjoint therapy, conjugal therapy.
Marriage therapy in which both partners confer with the therapist in joint sessions.

Ehespaltung marital schism.
Disharmony and open disagreement between the marriage partners. Each partner is so wrapped up in his or her own problems that parental roles are impaired. This may be one of the causative factors of schizophrenia in children.

Eifersuchtswahn delusional jealousy.
Delusions of infidelity entertained by one of the marriage partners. The partner affected is constantly on the watch for "evidence" to support his suspicions. The reaction is paranoid in nature and was once called *amorous paranoia.*

einfache Erinnerungsfälschung memory falsification.
The fictitious "recall" of events, usually in a boastful, bragging manner, in great detail. Like *confabulation,* the term is associated with KORSAKOFF's syndrome. The two English terms are almost identical, a possible difference being that confabulation is often held to be an attempt on the part of the patient to cover up his embarrassment about memory gaps. It is also associated with other organic psychoses.

Einfall sudden idea.
JUNG's term **freier Einfall** has been translated by *free association* since it is often considered to be very near to → **freie Assoziation.**

Einfluss → **prägende Einflüsse.**

Einfühlung empathy.
Awareness of another's feelings, volition, ideas and possibly of their interpretation. The person who empathizes, however, retains his objectivity and separate feelings.

eingebildete Schwangerschaft false pregnancy; hysterical pregnancy, pseudocyesis, spurious pregnancy, pseudopregnancy.
A rare condition in which a woman imagines she is pregnant. Most of the characteristics are indeed present – "everything except the baby".

Eingebung → **Gedankeneingebung.**

Einheitspsychose unitary psychosis.
Of historical interest only: GRIESINGER's view that all mental disorders were the expression of a single entity.
Ref.: Oxford Textbook of Psychiatry [6], p. 235.

Einschlafdenken hypnagogic reverie.
Fantasies occurring on the edge of sleep.

Einschlafstörungen initial insomnia.
Difficulty in falling to sleep owing to tension, anxiety or depression. Inability to "switch off" **(abschalten)** may also be due to worry about not sleeping. → **Bettangst.**

Einschlafzeremoniell sleep rituals.
"Ceremonies" necessary for some individuals as a preparation for sleep. The term belongs to the many rituals carried out as a defense

against anxiety or in order to release tension. FREUD gives the example of a boy who could not sleep until he had recited all the events of the day to his mother, pushed his bed to the wall and arranged three chairs against it. In this respect, *ritual* is employed by psychiatrists in rather a different way than by anthropologists and ethnologists.

Einsicht insight.
1. Awareness of underlying or unconscious origins of emotional difficulty; essential to psychotherapy. **2.** The patient's realization that his fears or obsessions are abnormal. Sometimes equated with the *aha experience* – the moment of sudden insight.

Einstellung attitude (in a general sense); mental set or rather inflexible attitude.
When employed in the latter sense, the German word is sometimes retained in English. → **motorische Einstellung.**
Ref.: Longman [7].

Einstellungstypen attitude types.
A Jungian term for the basic extraverted and introverted types. → **extravertierter Typus**, → **introvertierter Typus,** → Figures 4 and 5.

Einteilung → **topische Einteilung der Psyche** → Figure 2.

Einweisung admission (to a hospital) → **Zwangseinweisung.**

Einzelfallhilfe social case work; casework.
Social work involving consideration of the personal problems, needs, and relationships of an individual.

Einzelfallstudie case study; case study method.
An investigation carried out on detailed case histories and all other data with a view to shedding light on the individual's behavior and problems.

Ellbogen-Gesellschaft smash-and-grab society.
A form of capitalism said to be "without heart" by some, and by others as giving way to "caring capitalism".
Ref.: Kapitalismus ohne Herz. Frankfurter Allgemeine Zeitung, 23 April 1986.

Emotion emotion.
Generally synonymous in German and English, but SIFNEOS reserves the word to describe the biological side of *affect.* Expressed by behavioral means and mediated through the limbic system via the hypothalamus, it has a direct effect on the endocrine system and the autonomic nervous system, thus playing a key role in the exchange between the body and the outside world. → **Affekt,** → **Gefühl.**
Ref. → **Alexithymie.**

emotionaler Analphabetismus emotional inarticulateness.
This state refers to a type of ulcer patient and does not infer illiteracy in the usual sense. These patients repress disappointment and aggression resulting from lack of care and protection so as not to compromise their chances of obtaining moral support from their milieu.

emotionelle Mangelsituation emotional deprivation.
Lack of care and affection by the mother in early years, particularly in cases of separation. This may impair later emotional and intellectual development, and lead to maladjustment problems and even depression.

Emotionsstupor emotional stupor.
A state of stupor induced by frightening or catastrophic events, and accompanied by depressive symptoms and intense anxiety that render the victim incapable of speech.

Empfindung → **Gefühlsempfindung.**

Empfindungstypus → **extravertierter Empfindungstypus,** → **introvertierter Empfindungstypus.**

Empirismus empiricism.
A view that all science, including psychology, should be based on experience through the senses and introspection. Philosophically speaking, there are various forms and schools. Extreme empiricists confine our knowledge to statements about sense data, while others include analytic statements. *British empiricists* is the label for LOCKE, BERKELEY, and HUME, as well as for others sharing their outlook.

emsige Apathie "busy apathy".
The expression stems from KÜTEMEYER and denotes a bustling yet aimless activity of some older people who refuse to acknowledge their past for what it was. Such activity constitutes a form of distraction and prevents retrospection.

Enantiodromie enantiodromia.
Heraclitus' proposition that all things eventually turn into their opposites was employed by JUNG with respect to certain psychic processes, one example being the interplay between the conscious and the unconscious. He emphasized the need to become aware of one's own inner polarities.

Endlust end pleasure.
The release of tension during orgasm.
cf. **Vorlust** (forepleasure).

Enquête-Kommission
A commission set up by the West German Bundestag (Lower House) in 1971 to inquire into the state of psychiatric services in the Federal Republic.

Entäusserungshemmung inhibition of vocal expression.

Entfaltung development (e.g. of personality); display or exhibit abilities; burgeoning (in the sense of suddenly flourishing).

Entfremdung alienation (when breakdown of relationships is meant).
Both the German and English terms can refer to mental illness in general, but the German may also refer to depersonalization (→ **Wirklichkeitsentfremdung**).

Entgegenkommen → **somatisches Entgegenkommen.**

Enthemmung disinhibition.
Loss of control by the higher centers of the brain over the lower owing to brain damage or drugs. This may result in acute regressed behavior, since the lower centers are no longer inhibited. *Disinhibition* can also mean the revival of an extinguished conditioned reflex by a stimulus to which an experimental animal is unaccustomed.

Entkernung der Persönlichkeit personality deterioration.
The English term refers to a progressive loss of self-esteem, motivation, and sense of personal identity. The patient's emotional life diminishes to such an extent that he almost becomes a "nonperson". The German term employed by BRÄUTIGAM largely concurs with this definition except that this author gives the cause for the personality change as drug addiction. According to KIELHOLZ the condition is a consequence of long-term abuse of drugs or alcohol. The German term was coined by JOHN STAEHELIN and first used in relation to addiction by KIELHOLZ.

Entladung discharge (either emotional or electrical). → **Affektentladung.**

Entmachtung → **Selbstentmachtung.**

Entmischung defusion.
Reversal of the fusion of instincts that usually

Entmischung defusion.
Reversal of the fusion of instincts that usually accompanies maturity. This may occur in regression and lead to the separation of destructive/aggressive instincts from those of constructive, sexual instincts and result in perversions.

Entspannungstherapie relaxation training; relaxation therapy; body therapies.
Relaxation training usually refers to such techniques as autogenic training and progressive relaxation, whereas *relaxation therapy* relates more to differential relaxation (e.g. relaxing the left hand while using the right), and to muscle relaxants. *Body therapies* include most of the physical techniques for relieving tensions and other symptoms, e.g. breathing exercises, massage, manipulation, and postural exercises.

Entstellung distortion.
The modification of psychic content in order to make it acceptable to the ego. FREUD considered that the distortion occurring in an otherwise rational dream content was an example of taking over the idea by unconscious wishes at the preconscious stage. *Example:* a person's dream of rushing up the stairs will pass superego censorship easier than, say, the act of intercourse that it may represent. Similarly, some people give a warped account of an experience that would put them in a bad light. Pathologically speaking, many psychiatric symptoms may be distortions of mental processes.
Ref.: Longman [7]; ENCYCLOPAEDIA OF PSYCHIATRY FOR GENERAL PRACTITIONERS [8]; PETERS [11].

Entwicklungshomosexualität natural homosexual period; homosexual tendencies during the late latency stage.
The second term is nearer to the German but it is more of a definition than a widely accepted expression. *Natural homosexual period* is, however, sometimes applied in English to the stage when young people seek friends of the same sex, have "crushes" on each other and even on teachers of the same sex.

Entwicklungspsychologie developmental psychology.
A branch of psychology that deals with mental and other aspects of maturation, particularly in younger people.

Entwicklungsstadien stages of development. → **psychosexuelle Entwicklungsstadien.**

Entwicklungsstörung developmental disability; developmental disorder.
Any disorder acquired before adulthood which may influence future life. **Massive Entwicklungsstörungen** *pervasive developmental disorders.* This is the general term given to severe mental disorders in childhood. *DSM-III* lists numerous other categories.
cf. **geistige Behinderung,** → **trisomal-dysmorphe Entwicklungsstörung.**

Entwöhnungskur detoxification; rehabilitation (to more stable habits and ultimately to abstinence); "drying out".
There is no true English equivalent to the German term, since *weaning* **(Entwöhnung)** generally applies to infants being gradually given solid foods. It is a pity that the term *gradual dehabituation* has not been coined, since it would fill the bill admirably. *Rehabilitation* is sometimes used on its own when the meaning is clear from the context. Some authors speak of *withdrawal programs,* which may best be set up in a hospital or center. → **Entziehungskur;** → **Trinkerheilanstalt.**

Entwurzelung uprooting.
Generally, immigration to a strange country with a different culture, language, or environment. This may produce an *uprooting neurosis* or *uprooting psychosis.* In German, the term **Entwurzelungsdepression** comes very close to the *concentration camp syndrome* → **KZ-Syndrom.**

Entziehungserscheinungen withdrawal symptoms; withdrawal; abstinence syndrome.
The first two English terms are often interchangeable but *withdrawal* is, strictly speaking, the disorder brought about by discontinuing or severely reducing the intake of a drug or alcohol. The symptoms vary in accordance with the substance, but generally include irritability, restlessness, and insomnia. For possible ambiguity of the English term. *cf.* **Rückzug.**

Entziehungskur detoxification.
The German term is often equated with → **Entwöhnungskur**, though, strictly speaking, the latter should infer a gradual withdrawal from the drug, as is usually the case in treating barbiturate addiction. Alcohol, on the other hand, is withdrawn abruptly. Some authors speak of a *withdrawal program.*

Entzug withdrawal (of drugs or alcohol). → **Alkoholentziehungskur,** → **Entziehungskur.**

Episode → **psychogene psychotische Episode.**

erarbeiten to acquire (usually by work).
Etwas schwer erarbeiten to work hard for something.

Erbrechen vomiting. → **Zwangserbrechen.**

Erfahrung und Erlebnis → **Erlebnis** for differences in usage. *cf.* also **Selbsterfahrung.**

Erfahrungswissen empirical knowledge; practical knowledge. → **Empirismus.**

Ergasie ergasia.
A term introduced by Adolf Meyer (about 1904) describing integrated psychological, biological and social activities. *Ergasiology* is synonymous with *psychobiology*.

Erhaltungstherapie maintenance therapy.

Erinnerungsassoziation associative memory.
Recall to memory of an event or fact by virtue of something associated with it. The therapist may note key words used by a patient, which he then uses to establish *associative linkages.*

Erinnerungsausfall → **inselförmiger Erinnerungsfall.**

Erinnerungsfälschung memory distortion.
Inaccurate recall, usually unconsciously, of past events. This may occur in normal health, as, for example, in the case of witnesses in a court of law. An uncompromisingly unconscious distortion of memory in order to please others and conform to their expectations is termed *retrospective falsification.* When the conviction is held that events merely described have actually been witnessed or experienced, one speaks of *paramnesia.* → **positive Erinnerungsfälschung.**

Erinnerungsspur engram, memory trace, mnemonic trace, mneme.
A latent memory picture. In psychology it is a lasting trace left in the psyche by anything experienced emotionally. The term *engram* was first used in a neurological context by K. S. Lashley in 1950. Eccles maintained that the hippocampus, although not the seat of engrams, is the necessary instrument for laying them down, presumably in the cerebral cortex.
Ref.: Popper, K. R., Eccles, J. C.: The Self and Its Brain. Springer, Berlin–New York–London 1977.

Erinnerungsverlust amnesia, loss of memory. → **transitorische globale Amnesie.**

Erkennen cognition (in a philosophical sense).
Knowledge, awareness, and perception of facts. *cf.* **Konation.**

Erkenntnistherapie (Lungwitz) cognitive therapy (Beck); cognitive behavior therapy.

Treatment based on the correction of faulty ways of thinking. A philosophical approach. The modern trend is to use **kognitive Therapie** in German too.

erklären to explain.
The translation presents no problem, but it should be borne in mind that in the sense in which it was used by JASPERS the term refers to a scientific, causal explanation of, say, a patient's behavior (e.g. a specific organic cause) rather than intuitive understanding (*cf.* **Verstehen**).
Ref.: Oxford Textbook of Psychiatry [6], p. 86.

Erlebnis event; adventure; a moving or poignant experience.
These terms are not in any order of preference, since a choice would depend on the context. The difference between **Erlebnis** and **Erfahrung** is rather subtle. As a rule of thumb, the former may have a more emotional quality, while the latter is usually more factual and involves learning (→ **Erfahrungswissen**). **Erlebnisbedingt** can, for example, mean *psychogenic* in the right context, while **erfahrungsgemäss** is simply *from experience, according to experience,* or *empirically*.
→ **Aha-Erlebnis,** → **leibliches Beeinflussungserlebnis,** → **Urerlebnis.**

Erlebnisbeobachtung introspection.
Examination of one's own feelings and thoughts, sometimes in relation to sensory and perceptual experience. This is made use of in the *introspective method* (**Erlebnispsychologie**). → **Rückschau.**

Erlebnisreaktion emotional response (to an event or to a person).

Erlebnisweise pattern of subjective experience.

Erregung agitation.
A state of restlessness arising from tension and anxiety. *cf.* **Jammer-Depression.** *Psychomotor agitation* (**psychomotorische Erregung**) is similar but stems from subjective and emotional causes; mental overactivity is more pronounced. *Excitement* can be used when impulsive behavior or general arousal is involved. **Sexuelle Erregung** is termed the *excitement phase* in the sexual-response cycle (**sexuelle Erregungskurve**). ICD-9 lists the term *reative excitation* in relation to affective psychosis. *Excitation,* however, may in neurology refer to the activity in a nerve when stimulated.
cf. **Gefühlserregbarkeit.**

Ersatz → **Muttersatz.**

Ersatzbefriedigung substitution.
The replacement of a goal that is unattainable or unacceptable (to the superego) by alternative satisfactions. Similar to sublimation (**Sublimierung**).

Erschöpfungsdepression exhaustion depression.
The term was coined by KIELHOLZ. The condition occurs as a result of prolonged affective strain and usually goes through three stages: in the asthenic, hyperesthetic stage patients are irritable and sensitive; in the second stage, psychosomatic symptoms such as headaches appear; true depressive symptoms occur only in the third stage, with exhaustion of the adrenergic nervous system at the somatic level.

Erwartungsneurose performance neurosis.
A state in which anxiety is so intense that it may prevent carrying out a given task. Typical situations in which this occurs are public appearances and examinations.

Erziehungsberatungsstellen child guidance clinics. → **Kinderberatung.**

Es id.
The realm of the unconscious, of vital forces, and of instinctual biological drives. It sup-

ports and influences the ego **(Ich)** and superego **(Über-Ich).**

essen to eat. → **Rauschesser.**

Esstaumel binge; period of voracious eating.

ETB = Encephalopathia traumatica der Boxer → **Boxerenzephalopathie.**

Eviratio eviration.
RICHARD VON KRAFFT-EBING's term for emasculization and feminization. The verb is *to evirate.* In psychiatry, eviration refers to a delusional state in certain males that may be irreversible.

existentielle Angst existential anxiety.
This relatively recent category comes closest to KIERKEGAARD's concept of anxiety: a general fear of not being able to master this existence. Psychologically speaking, this would be the fear of self-realization.

Existenzangst existential anxiety.
The German term is in essence the same as → **existentielle Angst,** except that it is on a "higher" plane. Here there is a feeling of the impending destruction of one's existence, a dread of the void, as well as inability to perceive any meaning to life, coupled with the sense of alienation.
Ref.: Longman [7], entries "existential vacuum" and "Angst".

extravertierter Denktypus extraverted (extroverted) thinking type.
One of JUNG's basic functional types (→ Fig. 4) characterized by the tendency to shape his life and that of his family according to rigid rules. The mode of thought is positive, dogmatic and involves synthesis. *cf.* **introvertierter Denktypus.**

extravertierter Empfindungstypus extraverted (extroverted) sensation type.
One of JUNG's basic functional types (→ Fig. 4) characterized by a tendency to pleasure seeking, being sociable, and adapting to people and situations. *cf.* **introvertierter Empfindungstypus.**

extravertierter Fühltypus extraverted (extroverted) feeling type.
One of JUNG's basic functional types (→ Fig. 4) characterized by the tendency to cling to traditional values, respect social conventions, and be very emotional. *cf.* **introvertierter Fühltypus.**

extravertierter intuitiver Typus extraverted (extroverted) intuitive type.
One of JUNG's basic functional types (→ Fig. 4), characterized by a tendency to show insight into life situations and to enjoy finding out things. People of this type usually have a gift for business and politics. *cf.* **introvertierter intuitiver Typus.**

extravertierter Typus extraverted type.
JUNG's term for a person whose interests and modes of behavior are directed habitually outwards to other people and the physical environment. Such an individual is supposed to be sociable, active, and impulsive. *cf.* **introvertierter Typus,** → Fig. 5.

F

Fähigkeit ability. capability, competence. *cf.* → **Ehefähigkeit,** → **Geschäftsfähigkeit,** → **Geschäftsunfähigkeit,** → **Merkfähigkeit,** → **Reproduktionsfähigkeit.**

Faktor-X x factor.
Factors other than psychological, such as constitutional or acquired features which are present at the time of a disease. Organ vulnerability.

Fall case. → **Einzelfallhilfe,** → **Einzelfallstudie.**

familiäres Unbewusstes familial unconscious.
SZONDI's term for that part of the unconscious dominated or influenced by one's family history or ancestors, particularly in the choice of friends but also other preferences and behavior. → Fig. 2.

Fantasien → **Phantasien.**

Faseln drivel; rambling.
Colloquial expression for → **Weitschweifigkeit.**

Fehlhaltung 1. maladjustment.
Failure to achieve emotional harmony with one's surroundings and maintain relationships with people. This is also a vague term in English covering many minor emotional disturbances. Applied to children, *maladjustment* may refer to the result of harmful influences of individuals, deprivations, or a broken home.
2. faulty attitude.
Distortions engendered by prejudice, superstitions or aversions.
3. faulty posture or postural anomaly (in the orthopedic sense) = **Haltungsfehler.**
4. wrong position (of the fetus in obstetrics).

Fehlleistung parapraxis.
Symptomatic acts that may express unconscious desires. These include slips of the tongue, forgetfulness in important matters, and motivated accidents.

Fehlverhalten behavior disorder; behavioral disturbances.

Feldtheorie des Verhaltens field theory (of behavior).
LEWIN's theory that personal behavior could be deduced from a topological survey of one's "life space", particularly with respect to positive and negative *valences* (→ **Aufforderungscharakter**).

Fieberdelir; Fieberpsychose febrile delirium.
A mental disturbance marked by confusion and restlessness brought about by fever.

Fingerspitzengefühl intuition, flair, tact, sensitivity.
(All of which may sometimes be needed to select the English equivalent). **Hierfür braucht man Fingerspitzengefühl** could mean *this requires flair* but also *tact* in some circumstances (though *tact* is more **Feingefühl**).

Fixierung fixation.
The propensity to preserve patterns of behavior, feelings and ideas that have served well in the past. Yet persistent concentration on earlier libidinal desires, for example, may be unhealthy. The point of fixation determines the neurosis that develops in later life. A simplified way of stating the difference between *fixation* and *regression* would be: in fixation one "gets stuck" (in development); in regression one goes back a stage (or more). In both languages a given aspect of psychological

development fails to proceed beyond a certain immature stage.
In psychiatric clinics the German expression may moreover, refer to bed restraint. The term is extended to the focusing of both eyes on an object, or from one object to another (reading). The verb is *to fix* (not to be confused with drug addict slang!) or *fixate,* which may also refer to the reinforcement of a habit until it has reached the stage of a fixation.

Flachheit → **Gefühlsflachheit.**

Flucht in die Krankheit flight into illness.
A term employed by ADLER for the development of "nervous" symptoms. Physical complaints of minor nature tend to be exaggerated by the patient as an unconscious means of avoiding stressful situations. Other English terms: *escape into illness, flight into disease.*

freie Assoziation, freies Assoziieren free association.
A technique employed in psychoanalysis in which patients are encouraged to abandon conscious control over their thoughts and say whatever comes into their minds, no matter how irrelevant or embarrassing this may appear. The aim is to release unconscious material that is inhibited or repressed.

freiflottierende Angst free-floating anxiety.
A vague, chronic apprehension unrelated to any specific object.

Freiheitspsychose discharge psychosis.
This is only a suggested translation, since the German term refers to emotional symptoms occurring on obtaining release after long internment in a camp or institution; long-term inmates so affected are incapable of normal interpersonal relationships and leaving the camp of their own accord. The term *pre-release anxiety state* may be used in the case of prisoners who fear being released and having to compete in the outside world. *Furlough psychosis* is acute schizophrenic behavior that affects some soldiers soon after commencing leave.

Fremdanamnese independent history (obtained from close relatives or friends of the patient).

Fressgier; Fressucht bulimia.
Excessive and uncontrolled eating. → **Esstaumel.**

Freudscher Versprecher; Freudsches Versprechen Freudian slip. → **Fehlleistung.**

Friedreichsche Erinnerungskrämpfe → **Tourette Störung.**

Fortlaufen poriomania.
An irresistible impulse to run away from home. This is a simplification, since definitions do not fully coincide in both languages. In German, **Fortlaufen** in the sense of **Poriomanie** refers mostly to children leaving home, whereas in English *poriomania* implies the possibility of amnesia, and is regarded largely as a condition in senile and epileptic patients. This is essentially identical with the English use of *fugue,* but not with the German (which is synonymous with **Poriomanie**). → **psychogenes Weglaufen.**

Fugue → **Fortlaufen,** → **psychogenes Weglaufen.**

Fühltypus → **extravertierter Fühltypus,** → **introvertierter Fühltypus.**

funktionelle Blindheit → **psychogene Blindheit.**

funktionelle Psychose functional psychosis.
A disorder in which organic disorders play no part. Examples may be schizophrenia and manic depression, which are thought to stem from psychogenic factors. → **Funktionspsychose.**

funktionelle sexuelle Störungen psychosexual disorders.
Disorders of sexual function originating from psychological rather than organic factors, and including gender identity, paraphilias and disturbances in sexual response.

Funktionspsychose transient organic psychotic condition.
The German term stems from H. H. WIECK and includes all psychoses having organic causes that are reversible. One of the main features is clouded consciousness. The German term may also be confusing since it is sometimes used as a synonym for → **funktionelle Psychose.**
Ref.: German: PETERS [11]; English: Mental Disorders (Glossary) WHO 1978 [9], p. 25.

Funktionstypen → Fig. 4.

Furcht fear, dread, fright.
Fear is a signal response to an external danger that is actually present. Unlike anxiety (→ **Angst**), it is usually proportionate to the danger involved and often associated with the wish to fight or flee.

G

Ganser-Syndrom → **Gefängnispsychose.**

Ganzheit holism.

A philosophic notion that the whole is greater than the sum of its parts. This has given rise to such approaches as *holistic psychology,* one of the basic tenets of which is that healthy human development consists of mobilizing one's full potentialities and expressing them. Emphasis is placed on the integration of biological, psychological, and sociocultural factors, which cannot be fully explained in terms of individual facets. Likewise, *holistic medicine* is based on the premise that illness may affect the "whole man", including mind as well as body. The above is a simplification of a controversial term. Even its protagonist J. C. SMUTS employed the expression in two different ways. The brief definition of *holism* given here relates to EHRENFELS. Moreover, the term *holistic* has been taken over by certain faith-healing advocates.

Ref.:

1. PÖLDINGER, W.: Über systemisches und perspektives Denken in der Psychiatrie. Schweizerische Ärztezeitung 66, No. 29 (1985).

2. SMUTS, J. C.: Holism and Evolution. Macmillan, New York 1926.

3. EHRENFELS, CHR. VON: Über „Gestaltqualitäten". Vierteljahresschrift für wissenschaftl. Philosophie 14 (1890) 249–292.

Gedächtnis memory. → **Altgedächtnis,** → **biologisches Gedächtnis.**

Gedächtnisspanne memory span.

The number of items (digits, symbols, words, etc.) that an individual can reproduce correctly after one presentation. Tests of memory span are frequently employed in mental examinations. There are both *visual* and *auditory* memory spans.

Gedanken thought. → **Traumgedanken.**

Gedankenabreissen; Gedankenentzug thought withdrawal; delusions of thought withdrawal.

The patient has the impression that thoughts have been taken out of the mind by some external agency. This is given as an explanation by the patient for interrupted speech.

Ref. → **Gedankensperrung.**

Gedankenausbreitung thought-broadcasting.

A conviction, mainly of schizophrenic patients, that personal thought content is somehow being disseminated for others to hear.

Gedankenbeeinflussung constraint of thought.

A conviction, particularly in schizophrenic patients, that some external force is influencing or manipulating thought.

Gedankeneingebung thought pressure.

The feeling that external ideas are being forced into one's own mind. Characteristic of schizophrenia.

Gedankenlautwerden 1. écho des pensées; thought-echoing.

The patient has the auditory hallucination that his thoughts are repeated as a voice. He is aware that the thoughts are his own, and not some inner voice as in

2. audible thought. → **Doppeldenken.**

Gedankensperrung blocking.

An abrupt interruption of thought or speech flow. The process is unconscious and occurs particularly in schizophrenic patients, but it may take place with normal individuals in a transient form. The term is synonomous with *thought deprivation* and *thought obstruction.* *Ref.:* Oxford Textbook of Psychiatry [6]; SCHARFETTER, CHR.: Allgemeine Psychopathologie. Thieme, Stuttgart 1984.

Gefälligkeitstraum compliance dream.
A dream representing an unconscious desire to please the psychoanalyst and "confirm" his theories. A *made-to-order dream* has also been suggested.

Gefängnispsychose; Haftpsychose 1. prison psychosis.
An emotional breakdown in a prison setting. The clinical picture varies with the prisoner's former tendencies and character; it usually assumes paranoid forms, although depressive and delirious features may occur. It is sometimes regarded as simulated, but if untreated an impulsive attack on a warden or destruction may take place under the influence of delusions **(Haftknall).**
2. Ganser's syndrome.
Disturbances of memory which appear calculated to impress the observer with the prisoner's mental illness. Wrong answers to simple questions and hallucinations are also characteristic of the condition.

Gefahrenquotient (eines Arzneimittels) abuse liability.
The property of a substance to reinforce drug-taking behavior. Amphetamines have a high degree of abuse liability. The German term is sometimes employed for → **Risikoquotient.**

Gefühl feeling, sensation, touch.
Mostly *feeling* in psychiatric contexts. SIFNEOS contends that *feeling* should be reserved for the psychological side of *affect* and must contain the subjective fantasies and thoughts associated with it. Neocortical activity is a sine qua non – as opposed to *emotions.* → **Affekt,** → **Emotion.** *Ref.* → **Alexithymie.**
According to **Rohracher,** *feelings* are states that are inseparable from the other things a person is experiencing at the time, but which require an internal or external stimulus. They thus resemble drives, and occur without involvement of the conscious mind. → **Stimmung** (mood). Despite these delineations, **gefühlsbetont** is often equated with **affektbetont,** both of which may be translated by *emotional, with emotional overtones,* and the former (derogatory) by *sentimental* or *mawkish.* **Affektgeladen** may be rendered by *charged with emotion* or *laden with affect. cf.* **Fingerspitzengefühl,** → **Gemeinschaftsgefühl, Gefühl der Hilf- und Hoffnungslosigkeit,** → **Minderwertigkeitsgefühl,** → **Selbstgefühl,** → **Selbstwertgefühl.**

Gefühl der Hilf- und Hoffnungslosigkeit feelings of helplessness or hopelessness.
This is usually rendered in English by *giving up – given up complex,* which occurs in bereavement and depression (ENGEL).

Gefühlsansteckung contagion.
A psychosocial phenomenon in which ideas, doctrines, and types of behavior are disseminated from person to person or group to group. An extreme example is *mass hysteria.*

Gefühlsempfindung (STUMPF) sensation; feel.
Body sensations such as itching, tickling or stroking.

Gefühlserregbarkeit 1. emotional response.
This English term is restricted to the emotional reaction of people to events.
2. Excitability.
Generally speaking, the quality of being readily roused into action or excitement.
3. Sensibility.
The capacity to be stimulated; also, capacity for intense feeling.

Gefühlsflachheit 1. flat affect; emotional flatness.
Lack of emotional response to any situation or event. Common in schizophrenia.

2. emotional anesthesia.
Inability to react emotionally after repeated loss of one's fellows (→ **KZ-Syndrom**).

Gefühlslähmung 1. shock reaction.
An acute emotional disturbance immediately after a traumatic event. The victim is dazed and stunned, often unaware of the extent of his injury and may become stuporous.
2. disaster syndrome.
Similar to (1), but particularly after disasters. It has three stages: dazed, little help given to others; suggestible and passively dependent; tense and apprehensive.

Gefühlstheorie (JAMES und LANGE) James-Lange theory.
The theory of two independent investigators (about 1885) claiming that bodily changes, particularly vascular and visceral, come first, and give rise to emotional changes.

Gefühlstönung feeling tone.
→ **Stimmung.** Sometimes used to describe *affect* (→ **Affekt**).

Gegenbesetzung countercathexis, counter-investment, anticathexis.
The psychic energy employed by the unconscious to block id impulses entering into the conscious. Thus, countercathexis may be involved in concealing a tendency to hoard money or objects by acts of generosity to deserving causes. *cf.* → **Besetzung** (cathexis).

gegenphobische Aktivität counter-phobic activity; counterphobia.
Activity of a phobic individual representing an attempt to hide fears and even show courage and daring.

Gegensatzproblematik problem of opposites.
A problem which is profoundly characteristic of the psyche. The structure of the psyche is in fact so radically contradictory or contrapuntal that one can scarcely make any psychological statement without immediately having to state the opposite.
Ref.: JUNG, C. G.: Essays on Contempory Events. In [3].

Gegenübertragung countertransference.
The psychoanalyst's own repressed feelings are sometimes aroused by identifying himself with the patient's problems. This can impair his objective attitude towards the patient, but may provide extra insight. The negative aspect is usually taken care of in didactic analysis (→ **Lehranalyse**).

Gegenzwang countercompulsion.
A secondary compulsion intended to resist the original compulsion when it cannot be continued.

Geisteskrankheit mental illness; insanity.
In the broader sense, the German term refers to any form of mental illness. In the narrower sense it often refers to a psychosis or those forms that exhibit marked personality deviations, particularly schizophrenia. In English the terms at present most widely used are *mental illness* and *emotional disorders. Insanity* is more of a legal term, but there is a tendency to regard it as obsolete and replace it by *mental disorder.*

Geistesschwäche → **Schwachsinn.**

Geisteszustand mental status.
The English term refers to the psychological state of a person as shown by a mental examination. The German expression originates from legal parlance referring to the *state of mind* of a person at the time of committing a criminal act. Similarly, it is possible to say in English: "*mental capacity* to commit a crime requires the accused to know right from wrong" (WEBSTER).

geistige Behinderung; geistige Entwicklungsstörung mental retardation (the DSM-III term for *mental deficiency*).

A condition of arrested or incomplete development of mind which is especially characterized by subnormality of intelligence. The WHO lists several categories in English.
Ref.: WORLD HEALTH ORGANIZATION: Mental disorders [9].

Geltungstrieb striving for recognition.
The craving for acknowledgment of achievement by praise or awards. SCHULTZ-HENCKE rated this as one of the three major drives in man.

gemacht feeling of outside control (in schizophrenia); delusions of thought withdrawal and insertion (a first-rank symptom).

gemeinsame Gespräche joint round-table discussions (after MASTERS and JOHNSON).

Gemeinschaftsgefühl communal feeling; community spirit.
ADLER's expression hardly needs defining, but he rated such a feeling highly, and maintained that man could only realize his full potential as a member of society through good will and not with a "will to power" **(Wille zur Macht).** *Cf.* → **Machtstreben.**
Ref.: ALEXANDER: History of Psychiatry, p. 293.

Gemüthaftigkeit emotional responsiveness.

Gemütsarmut lack of emotional response.

Gemütsbewegung → **Emotion.**

Gemütskrankheit affective disorders.
The German term is vague but intended to differentiate disorders otherwise known as → **Geisteskrankheiten.** In the main it refers to endogenous depression and manic-depressive disorders (bipolar disorders).

Generalisierung → **Reizgeneralisierung.**

Generationentrennung generation gap.

gereizte Manie delirious mania.
An extreme state of mania marked by overactivity, screaming, querulous and aggressive behavior. Now rare owing to administration of psychotropic drugs.

Geruchshalluzination olfactory hallucination.
False perception of unpleasant odors; sometimes associated with guilt.

Gesamtdiagnose overall diagnosis.
A term originated by M. BALINT describing the diagnosis that is centered on the "whole man", embracing his psychological, social, and character-related conflicts.

Geschäftsfähigkeit competence.
Ability to understand the nature of a transaction and assume legal responsibility.

Geschäftsunfähigkeit incompetence.
Inability to make normal judgments in business transactions or assume responsibility. Hence, *incompetency plea.*

Geschlechtsidentität gender identity.
A sense of satisfaction or identification with the role and characteristics of one's own sex.

Geschlechtstrieb sexual instinct.
In psychoanalysis one also speaks of the term in the plural – sexual instincts – meaning all erotic drives and their sublimations. → **Trieb.**

Geschmackshalluzination gustatory hallucination.
A false taste, such as in imagining food is poisoned.

Gesellschaft → **Ellbogen-Gesellschaft,** → **Leistungsgesellschaft.**

Gesellschaftstrieb social instinct.
The tendency for individuals to engage in group activities or otherwise congregate. In psychoanalysis it is considered a basic urge,

beginning with parents and siblings and later extending to wider units.

Gesetz der Sparsamkeit law of parsimony; Morgan's canon.
When several hypotheses exist to explain a phenomenon, the most likely to be correct is the simplest or that requiring the least number of prior assumptions.
Ref.: Neel [10a], p. 28; [10b], p. 51.

Gesichtsfeld field of vision; perception.
Example: **die Einengung des Gesichtsfeldes auf das rein physiologische:** restriction of perceptions to purely physiological aspects.

Gespräche → gemeinsame Gespräche.

Gesprächstherapie 1. interview therapy.
This is the general term for every systematic type of dialogue influencing the course of the disorder in a positive manner, i.e. helping patients to resolve their problems or adjust to them, and even get to the roots of their conflicts.
2. Client-centered therapy.
This more specific term is used when referring to the nondirective approach of Carl Rogers. The therapy is aimed at encouraging the patient to develop his own inner potentialities. Although the patient arrives at his own interpretations in solving the problems, the therapist helps in self-perception. Unlike psychoanalytic therapy, the nondirective approach excludes the concept of the unconscious.

Gestaltkreis perceptual feedback; morpho-psycho-psychological circle.
A term used by V. von Weizsäcker describing how the reciprocal relationship between the organism and its surroundings is that of a functional whole. In walking over uneven ground, for example, the eyes note every irregularity, to which the body adapts its movements and in turn directs the gaze.

Gestaltpsychologie gestalt psychology.
A theory focusing on the investigation of how perceptual experience is organized into configurations **(Gestalten)** which cannot be split up. This property is called the *quality of configuration* **(Gestaltqualität).** The essence is that the whole is more important than the sum of its parts – as shown by the simple experiment that lights flashed successively give the impression of motion.

Gestalttherapie gestalt therapy.
Derived from gestalt psychology, the treatment focuses on constantly leading the patient back to his "here and now" relationships and abilities in their totality. Investigation into past experiences or the interpretation of dreams is not performed. The treatment is intended to encourage the patient's spontaneous feelings and promote self-awareness. Different techniques are employed, including acting out (→ **agieren**) and role-playing. It is an experiential rather than a verbal or interpretive therapy.

Gestaltungstherapie 1. art therapy.
The expression of conflicts and problems by artistic activities. No particular artistic ability is required and the choice of activity is wide, e.g. painting, modelling, dancing, etc.
2. occupational therapy.
Employing the patient in useful activities such as handicrafts. This type of therapy is now directed more toward active rehabilitation than mere diversion. → **künstlerische Gestaltungstherapie.**

Geständniszwang a compulsion to confess.
This arises, for example, when an individual is more afraid of his own inner moral judgement than of a court of law.

Getriebenheit compulsive behavior.

Gewissensangst moral anxiety.
This arises when we have the inclination to

infringe on certain precepts that we have been taught to keep.

Gewöhnung habituation.
The usage of this term varies in accordance with the particular discipline and context. In general, it denotes the process of growing accustomed to a situation or pattern of behavior. For the psychologist and psychiatrist it is the process of becoming psychologically dependent on the use of a particular drug, such as cocaine, but without the increasing tolerance and physiological dependence that are so characteristic of addiction (→ **Sucht**). It may also refer to the elimination of side responses by repetition that interfere with learning a skill. For the pharmacologist, habituation is progressive adaptation of the organism to ever increasing amounts of a stimulus or drug. As a result of increased tolerance, continually higher doses are necessary in order to achieve the same effect. *cf.* **Tachyphylaxie.**

Gewohnheitshierarchien habit hierarchies.
The arrangement of simpler habits into more complex patterns. This is often disturbed in schizophrenia.

gezielte Analyse focussed analysis.
A form of psychotherapy in which only a specific part of the patient's problems is subjected to interpretation.

glucksend gurgling.
Example: **glucksende Geräusche im Bauch:** gurgling noises in the stomach. (A description given by many patients of their symptoms; by "stomach" they may mean abdomen.)

Granatschock shell shock.
Both terms relate to World War I. For modern terms → **Kriegsneurose.**

Grenzbereich borderline.
The term *borderline* is also used in German to describe types of neurosis and psychosis. However, in the German translation of *DSM-III,* **Grenzbereich der Intellektuellen Leistungsfähigkeit** will be found for *borderline intellectual functioning:* an IQ between 71 and 84. Commonly called *borderline intelligence.*

Grössen-Selbst grandiose self.
H. Kohut developed a "self" theory that challenged Freud's. The term refers to the original narcissism in the child and is largely identical with the psychoanalytic expression *primary narcissism.*

Grössenwahn delusions of grandeur.
A grossly exaggerated and often distorted conception of one's own importance, power, and influence.

Grossvater-Komplex grandfather complex.
The desire of a male child to become his own grandfather, i.e. his parents' parent.

Grübelzwang rumination.
Persistent brooding or meditation on a problem. A common symptom of obsessive-compulsive disorders.

Grundsymptome fundamental symptoms.
Bleuler's term distinguishing primary from secondary symptoms in schizophrenia. They comprise autism, ambivalence, schizophrenic dementia, disturbances in attention, activity, and of associations.

Gruppe → **Hausgruppe.**

Grusskrämpfe → **Blitz-Nick-Salaam-Krämpfe.**

H

Haftknall impulsive act of a prisoner. → **Gefängnispsychose.**

Haftpsychose → **Gefängnispsychose.**

Halluzination → **Geruchshalluzination,** → **Geschmackshalluzination,** → **Tasthalluzination**

Haltung posture, attitude. → **anerkennende Haltung,** → **Fehlhaltung.**

Haltungsveränderungen postural changes.

Handlung → **Übersprungshandlung.**

Häufigkeitsquotient *Syn.* **Prävalenz** prevalence.
The total number of cases of a disease existing at a given point in time in a given area, usually expressed per 100,000 population.

Hausgruppe cooperative urban house (group).
A group of patients in a residence where they can still have certain supervision, yet be given some responsibilities, work, and take part in group activities. The more general term for this facility is a *halfway house.*

Heautoskopie autoscopic syndrome; autoscopy; autoscopic phenomenon.
A disorder in which the patient has the delusion of seeing a person who looks and acts like himself (though this may be very vague or hazy). If there is evidence of an organic basis for the disorder it is called *symptomatic autoscopy,* and *idiopathic autoscopy* if psychogenic. *cf.* **Doppelgängererlebnis.**

Heilanstalt psychiatric hospital, mental home, sanatorium, asylum. → **Trinkerheilanstalt.**

Heilpädagogik special education.
Education for children with learning or other disabilities, e.g. mental retardation, speech impairment, blindness, etc.

Hilfe → **Einzelfallhilfe.**

Hierarchie hierarchy. → **Angsthierarchie,** → **Gewohnheitshierarchien.**

Hemmung → **Entäusserungshemmung,** → **Enthemmung.**

Hilf- und Hoffnungslosigkeit → **Gefühl der Hilf- und Hoffnungslosigkeit.**

Hingabe devotion. → **Selbsthingabe.**

Hingabebedürfnisse und Versorgungswünsche a desire to care and be cared for, a desire to give and receive care.

Hirnleistungsschwäche cerebral dysfunction(s); impaired cerebral function.
Mental impairment usually associated with organic brain syndrome. Affected are memory, general intelligence, and consciousness.

Hoffnungslosigkeit → **Gefühl der** → **Hilf- und Hoffnungslosigkeit.**

Homosexualität → **Entwicklungshomosexualität.**

Hörigkeit compliance.
The German expression originally related to the services due from a tenant farmer to his proprietor, i.e. *bondage.* It now generally implies *emotional attachment to another person to the point of relinquishing personal freedom and dignity,* particularly in the sexual sphere. This largely coincides with *com-*

pliance when this English term denotes a readiness to yield to the demands of others, and particularly in the psychiatric sense where compliance is a *compulsion to yield* to the desires of others, when it sometimes reaches the stage of neurotic oversubmissiveness. It is unfortunate that *compliance* may also mean friendly agreement in a general sense, as well as positive cooperation of a patient with the doctor in the matter of taking drugs prescribed. Care must thus be observed with the context. Similarly, *bondage* is sometimes used to describe a voluntary subjugation or servitude to someone superior, but it now has the connotation of a form of mock enslavement in order to arouse sexual desire. A more literary rendering of **Hörigkeit** would be *to be in thrall to* (or *with*) someone (or something).

hypersensitive Persönlichkeitsstörung avoidant personality disorder.
A disorder occurring with a type of personality susceptible to extreme sensitivity with regard to rejection and humiliation. Demand for uncritical acceptance causes social withdrawal despite a strong desire for affection and recognition.

hysterische Blindheit → psychogene Blindheit.

hysterogene Punkte hysterogenic zones.
Areas of the body on which pressure or stimulation produces hysterical reactions such as pain or anesthesia. CHARCOT's idea of such circumscribed zones was largely rejected by FREUD.

I

Ich ego.
The ego is responsible for conscious parts of the personality, self-awareness and voluntary behavior; it is the organized part of the personality whereas the id (→ **Es**) is "unorganized" (→ Fig. 2).

Ich-Anachorese (nach WINKLER) extreme form of ego withdrawal.
The term refers to a retreat of the ego from incompatible conscious content, i.e. impulses from the id that are censored by the superego. It constitutes a dynamic explanation for the onset of schizophrenic symptoms.
Ref.: For full explanation see: SCHARFETTER, CHR.: Allgemeine Psychopathologie, S. 77. Thieme, Stuttgart 1984.

Ichbewusstsein ego consciousness.
Consciousness of the ego identity (→ **Ich-Identität**).

ichfremd ego-dystonic; ego-alien.
Adjective for ideas or impulses that are unacceptable to one's self or ego.

Ichgrenzen ego boundaries.
According to PAUL FEDERN, an inner boundary exists between the ego and the unconscious and an outer boundary between the ego and stimuli from the external world. The inner boundary prevents the entry of repressed material into the conscious mind, except under certain circumstances, e.g. while falling asleep. A feeling of unreality is produced when the outer boundary becomes permeable.

Ich-Identität ego identity
1. The unchanging consciousness of an individual about his identity, particularly with respect to what he was and is. In illness he may no longer be what he was.
2. Experience of the self as an entity by integrating one's ego ideal, life role in society, and adjustment to reality. This may be disturbed in hysteria and endogenous depression.

Ichlibido ego libido.
That part of the libido which is invested in one's own person (→ **Libidobesetzung**). It usually denotes the contrary to object libido. *Ego cathexis* is the preferred English term, although this is more the investment of psychic energy in the conscious ego. *cf.* **Objektlibido.**

Ichtriebe ego instincts.
Non-sexual instincts directed towards self-preservation, e.g. eating and defecating. The term stems from the earlier theory of instincts evolved by FREUD.

Ideenflucht flight of ideas; topical flight.
A thought disturbance in which there is an excess of basically unrelated and rapidly changing ideas. Thought is superficial and the thread is constantly lost. The condition is encountered in manic states and sometimes in schizophrenia.

Identifikation identification.
In psychoanalysis an unconscious process in which one would like to resemble someone else and behave in the same way. It is one of the ego defense mechanisms and is very similar to introjection, but less complete.

Identifizierung mit dem Angreifer identification with the aggressor.
ANNA FREUD's term for a defense mechanism by means of which a person may identify

himself with the behavior and other characteristics of an unbeatable opponent or enemy. It is similar to the *Stockholm syndrome,* in which hostages sometimes identify themselves with their captors, joining and even falling in love with them.

Identität → Geschlechtsidentität, → Ich-Identität.

Imponieren display; display behavior.
A type of behavior intended by one animal to attract the attention of another and elicit response. A kind of body language that may be used in courtship or as a show of power and aggression. "... quacks ... who flourished in the 18th century, then as now, by the kind of *bullying assurance* which the Germans call **imponieren**." (GARRISON).

Imponiergehabe demonstrative behavior.
Ref.:
1. LORENZ, KONRAD: Über tierisches und menschliches Verhalten. Piper, München 1984. (English translation: Studies in Animal and Human Behavior. Harvard University Press, Cambridge, Mass., 1971.)
2. MORRIS, DESMOND: The Naked Ape. Dell Press, New York 1984.

Indexpatient the presenting family member; sick individual family member; propositus. BALINT's → **Präsentiersymptom.**

induzierte paranoide Störung shared paranoid disorder (*DSM-III*); folie à deux, double insanity.
A disorder of a delusional character that is taken over from a person already affected by another owing to a close relationship. Despite the original French term, more than two persons may be involved. → **symbiontische Psychose → symbiotische Psychose.**

infaust unfavorable.

Inhalt content. → **Rauschinhalt,** → **Trauminhalt,** → **inhaltliche Denkstörungen**

inhaltliche Denkstörungen content-thought disorder.
Disturbances in thought content by delusions, bizarre ideas, and fragmentation. Characteristic of schizophrenia.

Initialschrei epileptic cry; initial cry.
The cry produced at the beginning of a grand mal seizure. It is caused by tonic contraction of the chest and laryngeal muscles.

inneres Mitmachen → Einfühlung.

innerseelischer Konflikt intrapsychic conflict.
Conflict evoked by impulses, ideas and emotions that arise within the individual's own mind or psyche. Unfortunately, the English term is sometimes used loosely for interpsychic conflict. *cf.* → **zwischenmenschlicher Konflikt.**

inselförmiger Erinnerungsausfall localized amnesia; lacunar amnesia; circumscribed amnesia.
Short gaps in memory restricted to specific periods, events or experiences.

Instinkt instinct; instinctual drive; instinctual impulse.
In both languages the term is eschewed by some specialists, and it is best avoided in a human medical context wherever possible. Some scientists restrict instinct to such animal faculties as "nestbuilding", while others may use the expression *self-preservation instinct* (→ **Selbsterhaltungstrieb**) in connection with man. This constitutes a problem for the translator, who should note the direction taken by the author. If it is in that taken by FREUD, McDOUGALL, and LORENZ, the term may still be used. Likewise, the German-speaking author should bear his readership in mind when employing the expression in an original article or dissertation written in English. → **Trieb.**

Intelligenzabbau intellectual deterioration; intellectual impoverishment.
The German term refers to the loss of inborn and acquired intelligence owing to age and disease. The first English term is rather more general, while the second also includes depletion in the level of interest as well as failing power to solve problems. Intellectual impoverishment may occur in schizophrenia, senility with depressive states, and in lack of environmental stimulus.

Intelligenzalter mental age (MA).

$$MA = \frac{\text{Intelligence test result of individual}}{\text{Average score for others of same age}}$$

(not applicable beyond 14 years of age).

internationale Kurznamen international nonproprietary names (INN). Two stages, 'proposed' and 'recommended', must be passed before final acceptance.

Intoxikationspsychose toxic psychosis.
A psychosis resulting from the ingestion of poisons. The symptoms are generally hallucinations, delirium, and restlessness.

Intratrachealkatheter endotracheal catheter.

Introjection introjection.
In psychoanalysis, the assimilation of other persons' standards or ideals into one's own ego or superego. One of the ego-defense mechanisms.

introvertierter Denktypus introverted thinking type.
One of JUNG's basic functional types (→ Fig. 4) characterized by a tendency to have little sense of practical issues and to isolation. Boldness and originality of ideas are largely inhibited by hesitation and scruples. *cf.* **extravertierter Denktypus.**

introvertierter Empfindungstypus introverted sensation type.
One of JUNG's basic functional types (→ Fig. 4) characterized by a tendency to be calm, while observing events with a mixture of benevolence and amusement. People of this type are often receptive to aesthetic qualities.
cf. **extravertierter Empfindungstypus.**

introvertierter Fühltypus introverted feeling type.
One of JUNG's basic functional types (→ Fig. 4), characterized by the tendency to be modest, quiet, oversensitive, and difficult to understand. The woman belonging to this type is said to exert an uncanny influence on extravert men.
cf. **extravertierter Fühltypus.**

introvertierter intuitiver Typus introverted intuitive type.
One of JUNG's basic functional types (→ Fig. 4), characterized by the tendency to be a day-dreamer attributing the greatest value to his own thoughts and feelings. People of this type are often regarded by others as being strange and eccentric. *cf.* **extravertierter intuitiver Typus.**

introvertierter Typus introverted type.
JUNG's term for a person who is inwardly directed to his own thoughts and feelings, and whose interests are theoretical rather than practical. Such an individual is held to be sensitive, contemplative, and reserved. *cf.* **extravertierter Typus,** → Fig. 5.

involutive Depression, *Syn.:* **Altersdepression. → Rückbildungsalter.**

Inzestschranke incest barrier.
The barrier arising during the latency period against impulses for sexual relationships with close relatives. The Freudian view is that this is culturally acquired through social laws and customs. *Incest taboo* refers more to a social

prohibition that is culture-dependent. "... bizarre extensions of incest groups ... the diverse ways in which different people have extended and elaborated the incest taboos ..." (MARGARET MEAD).

Ref.: MEAD, M.: Male and Female, p. 52. Penguin (1971).

Inzidenz incidence.
The number of new cases of a disease occurring during a given period (e.g. per year), usually given as per 100,000 population. *cf.* **Prävalenz.**

Isolierzelle seclusion room.
A room for isolating psychiatric patients who constitute a danger to other patients or are suicide risks. Also called the *isolation room,* and sometimes the *quiet room.*

J

Jacobsonsche Methode, *Syn.:* **Jacobsonsches Entspannungstraining** progressive relaxation.

A technique in which certain muscle groups are contracted, then relaxed progressively, also by conscious awareness. JACOBSON compiled a list of muscles to be employed in this technique. The method is used particularly in active desensitization.

Ref.: JACOBSON, E.: Progressive Relaxation. University of Chicago Press, Chicago 1938.
LUBAN-PLOZZA, B., PÖLDINGER, W.: Psychosomatic Disorders in General Practice, 2nd English edition, p. 142. Editiones Roche, Basle 1985.

Jammer-Depression, *Syn.:* **weinerlich-agitierte Depression, klagsam-agitierte Depression** agitated depression.

A type of depression in which the patient bemoans his fate, shows anguish, and is very restless. Also known as *ademonia.*

Jokaste-Komplex Jocasta complex.

An abnormal or neurotic attachment of a mother to her son. (Jocasta was the mother and later the wife of Oedipus).

Jugendkriminalität juvenile delinquency.

Unlawful behavior by minors: mostly vandalism, theft, assault, rape, and drug abuse.

jugendliche Paralyse juvenile paresis.

A form of general paresis occurring in children as a result of congenital syphilis. It is transmitted from mother to fetus during pregnancy, but the symptoms generally arise after the age of ten and include visual disorders, memory impairment and general deterioration.

K

Kampf oder Flucht fight or flight.
The expression stems from CANNON'S emergency theory of emotions: emotional and visceral changes controlled by the autonomic system prepare us for fight or flight. The term is usually contracted in such expressions as *fight-flight reaction.*

Kampfreaktion, → akute Kampfreaktion.

Kastrationsangst castration complex.

katathymes Bilderleben (KB) Guided Affective Imagery (GAI).
A psychotherapeutic technique in which daydreams and fantasies are encouraged and guided by the therapist. The method is employed in brief psychotherapy.

Katatonie catatonia. → **akute tödliche Katatonie.**

Katheter → Intratrachealkatheter.

Kernneurose neurotic nucleus.
J. H. SCHULTZ'S original expression has been defined as neurosis involving deeper levels of the personality, and that it is in many aspects identical with **Charakterneurose.** People with the latter structure are, moreover, particularly at risk under stress situations. *Neurotic nucleus* is also employed as a personality pattern giving rise to high vulnerability to stress and low frustration tolerance. In English, the term *character neurosis* is more of a condition in which such traits as overmeticulousness are part of a personality disorder rather than of a true neurosis. This term tends to be eschewed in Great Britain, where it has been held that "character" denotes moral judgement. A literal translation of **Kernneurose** to be avoided at all costs is "nuclear neurosis", which is a lay term for complaints of some people working in or around nuclear power plants!

Keuchen wheezing, wheeze.
→ **asthmatisches Keuchen.**

Kinderberatung child guidance.
In its formal setting of the "child guidance clinic" this is a service for the diagnosis, prevention, and treatment of behavioral and emotional disorders in childhood. Unlike child psychiatric departments in hospitals, the guidance clinics are usually situated in establishments closely linked to other community health and welfare facilities.

Kinderpsychose psychotic disorders in childhood.
Examples: childhood autism; neurotic disorders (rare); personality disorders; tics. "Childhood schizophrenia" is a debatable term.

kindliches Kopfwerfen (jactatio capitis nocturna) head-rolling.
Repetitive rolling of the head from side to side observed in some children just before going to sleep.

Kindsmisshandlung child abuse; battered-child syndrome.
The second term, which is more recent, refers to a pattern of abuse, usually by parents. It includes physical injury and neglect (emotional and nutritional).
"Child molestation" has more of a sexual or incestuous connotation.

klagsam-anklagend complaining-accusatory.
A type of behavior occurring, for example, on

object loss. A less literal translation: *complaining-cum-accusatory.*

Klangassoziationen clang associations; clanging.
Associations of words in accordance with their sounds rather than by their meaning. It is encountered in manic and schizophrenic disorders, but may be normal in childhood.

klares Bewusstsein full consciousness; full awareness; the state of being fully conscious.
The level of consciousness in normally healthy people. Other, psychopathological levels: *cf.* **Benommenheit,** → **Bewusstlosigkeit,** → **Bewusstseinstrübung.**

Kleinhirnanfall cerebellar fit.
Seizure with loss of consciousness due to a tumor of the vermis. Other symptoms are dilated pupils, cyanosis, and opisthotonos.

Klient client.
The term is often used in both languages instead of "patient" by social workers and counseling psychologists. → **Gesprächstherapie.**

klientenzentrierte Psychotherapie → **Gesprächstherapie.**

Klima → **affektives Klima.**

Knotenpunkt → **affektive Knotenpunkte.**

Koitusverbot abstention from intercourse.
The therapist imposes abstinence on the partners for a given time (but not on fondling or caressing) with the reverse intention.

Kollektiv (von Patienten) patient population.
Frequently this can be rendered simply by *patients.* However, if it refers to a number of patients taking part in an epidemiological study and sharing some statistical characteristic, *cohort* would be better.

kollektives Unbewusstes collective unconscious.
That part of the unconscious, which, according to JUNG, contains inherited elements common to large sections of mankind (hence the term *racial unconscious,* which is sometimes used in a restricted sense). → Fig. 2.

Koma coma; comatose state.
The deepest state of unconsciousness (the third and ultimate degree of clouding of consciousness (→ **Bewusstseinstrübung**). There is hardly any or no response to stimuli and an absence of reflexes.

Kommission → **Enquête-Kommission.**

Kommunikationstherapie 1. structural family therapy (MINUCHIN).
The role of the therapist is like that of a play director: to help the members of a family try out ways of communicating with one another, bringing to light unspoken rules by which they interact.
2. strategic therapy (HALEY).
Provoking the family into desirable actions and helping them set goals.
3. conjoint family therapy (SATIR).
The therapist's role is that of a teacher who instructs the members how to communicate.
All methods come under the main heading of *family therapy* and the sub-heading of *communication and systems methods. cf.* → **Systemtherapie.**
Ref.: Oxford Textbook of Psychiatry [6], p. 597.

kommunikative Resonance empathy, rapport.

Komplex → **Grossvater-Komplex,** → **Jokaste-Komplex,** → **Minderwertigkeitskomplex.**

Komplex-Bereitschaft "complex readiness".
A. A. BRILL's translation of BLEULER's original term, which referred to a state of mind in which a person tends to disclose a vulnerable point in his or her eagerness to conceal it.
Ref.: BRILL, A. A.: Basic Principles of Psychoanalysis [2].

komplexe Psychologie
→ analytische Psychologie.

Komponente → Versagungskomponente.

Konation conation.
Striving and action involving motives of all kinds. *Adj.: conative.*
→ Erkennen.

Konditionierung
→ operante Konditionierung.

Konflikt → Aversions-Aversions-Konflikt, → innerseelischer Konflikt, → psychischer Konflikt, → zwischenmenschlicher Konflikt.

konkretes Denken concrete thinking.
The second stage in the development of thought processes. Objects become recognized as either inanimate or animate, but no generalization or abstraction takes place: a table is seen as a specific table and not as one example of a whole range of such objects. It is encountered not only in children, but also in adult schizophrenic patients, and particularly in persons with frontal-lobe lesions. In normal children, this is the stage following syncretic thinking. **→ synkretes Denken.**
Ref.: Roche Encyclopaedia [8].

Konstanzprinzip law of constancy; principle of constancy (FREUD).
The principle that the sum of all mental processes and stimuli is held as constant as possible, i.e. it tends to reach a state of equilibrium or stability.

Konsumsitten consumer habits.

Kontakt → Blickkontakt.

Kontaktwahn induced insanity; folie à deux; shared paranoid disorder (*DSM-III*).
Delusions developing from contact with another person or other persons.

Kontrollanalyse controlled analysis.
Psychoanalysis performed by a candidate under the supervision of a fully qualified psychoanalyst.

Kontrolle → Realitätskontrolle.

Kontrollzwang obsessive doubt.
Uncertainty accompanied by excessive brooding and often by continual checking. It is encountered in obsessive-compulsive disorders, but may be present in very mild forms in normally healthy people.

Konversion conversion.
In psychosomatics synonymous in both languages. Repressed psychic material is transformed into somatic symptoms. The DSM-III term is *conversion disorders. Example:* a man may develop stiffness, or even paralysis, of the arm after repressing an impulse to strike someone. Unlike somatization, the physical form taken by the conflict is clearly symbolic. Moreover, the part of the body concerned is innervated by sensory or motor nerves. **→ Somatisierung, → Ausdruckskrankheiten, → Austragungsweisen.**

Konzeptionsfurcht fear of pregnancy.

Kopfschmerz(en) headache(s).
→ Spannungskopfschmerz.

Kopfuhr mental clock.
A mechanism or aptitude possessed by some people to wake up at the desired time without an alarm clock or similar device.

Kopfwerfen → **kindliches Kopfwerfen.**

Körperschema body image.
Knowledge of our own body and the way we view it. This picture is usually formed at an early age. When viewing its physical and functional attributes one speaks of *body concept,* and *body percept* when attitudes towards the body's characteristics are involved. When the body percept is derived from sensations of touch, posture or movements as well as structure one may speak of a *body schema* or *scheme.*

Körpertherapie body therapies.
The term is mostly employed in the plural in English, since it embraces all techniques that afford relief by manipulations, massage, breathing exercises and relaxation. Biofeedback and autogenic training are other examples.
N. B.: Somatic therapy is incorrect, since this infers treatment by electroshock, psychotropic drugs or other organic approaches.

Körperwerfen jactitation.
Tossing to and fro. → **kindliches Kopfwerfen.**

Kraftlosigkeit asthenia.

Krampf spasm (generally), convulsion, cramp, seizure.
There is much overlap between the first two terms in practical usage, though some authorities suggest *convulsion* is more severe, while even twitching may be classed as spasm. Important is that both are involuntary. *Examples: clonic spasm,* or *convulsion* – where rigidity is alternated with relaxation. *Tonic spasm,* or *convulsion* – where rigidity is sustained. The term *seizure* is preferred for epileptic convulsions. → **Blitz-Nick-Salaam-Krämpfe,** → **audiogene Krämpfe.** *Cramp* is used in such expressions as *writer's cramp* (**Schreibkrampf**) or other painful conditions. → **Friedreichsche Erinnerungskrämpfe,** → **Lachkrampf.**

Krankheit → **Flucht in die Krankheit** → **Geisteskrankheit,** → **Gemütskrankheit,** → **Managerkrankheit,** → **psychosomatische Krankheit.**

Krankheitsgewinn advantage by illness.
The exploitation of neurotic symptoms in order to gain sympathy and attention from the social milieu. In psychoanalysis this is called *epinosic gain,* or simply *epinosis. Primary gains* of this type present inner advantages, i.e. basic psychological advantages, by means of which the patient can avoid threatening situations. *Secondary gains* are concerned more with winning added attention, avoiding work, and even obtaining a pension. → **Flucht in die Krankheit** → **Assekurose.**

Krankheitswahn hypochondriasis, hypochondria.
A neurotic disorder. Excessive concern for health, integrity and function of the body, less frequently of the mind.

Kränkung offense, injury or mortification.

Kreuz → **psychosomatisches Kreuz.**

Kriegsneurose war neurosis.
A sequel to long exposure to wartime conditions. The German term is somewhat vaguer than the English, but both have conversion symptoms in common. The English term covers the tension produced by, say, severe bombardment and internal conflicts. There is some overlap with *combat fatigue.* → **Kampfreaktion.**

Kummernummer → **Telefonseelsorge**

Kummerspeck weight gain from overeating caused by worry.
The concise and picturesque German expression cannot be rendered in English unless some leading writer in the field of nutrition or psychiatry coins a new term, e.g. "worry-fat" or even "worry-belly".

künstlerische Gestaltungstherapie art therapy. → **Gestaltungstherapie.**

Kunstsprache neologistic jargon.
A form of speech in which the speaker coins his own idioms and terms, making his language difficult or impossible to follow. The juxtaposition of expressions is also inappropriate. *Agrammatism* is a type of aphasia in which the speech is so ungrammatical that it is incomprehensible. It is encountered more in Pick's and Alzheimer's disease than in schizophrenia.

Kur (course of) treatment; baths; spa treatment; taking the waters; cure.
→ **Alkoholentziehungskur**, → **Entwöhnungskur,** → **Redekur,** → **Schlafkur**

Kurzanalyse, Kurztherapie, short-term therapy.
Assistance with emotional problems and maladjustment over weeks rather than months. Such approaches may be applied on a deeper level, as in hypnoanalysis or narcosynthesis.

Kurznamen → **internationale Kurznamen.**

Kurzschlusshandlung intermittent explosive disorder.
An impulse control disorder, but unlike the isolated explosive disorder (**primitive Affektreaktion**) a series of outbursts is involved that usually results in serious damage to property, theft and perhaps suicide. Again, the acts are out of proportion to any stress present, as in the "isolated" variation, but the rational part of the personality is not entirely bypassed. → **primitive Affektreaktion.**

KZ-Syndrom concentration-camp syndrome.
A condition of constant anxiety, defenses against it, stress, and an obsessive ruminative state, possibly culminating in a form of reactive depression. In addition there is often "survival guilt" and self-protective response ("emotional anesthesia") toward those who died.

L

Lachen laughing. → **Zwangslachen.**

Lachkrampf (hysterischer) spasmodic laughter, gelasmus, hysterical laughter.
Persistent and uncontrollable laughing which may result in exhaustion. Despite the third term, it is also encountered in schizophrenia and in bulbar and pseudobulbar brain disease. *'Hysterical laughter'* used in a literary sense may not necessarily refer to a pathological state. → **Zwangslachen.**

Lähmung → **Gefühlslähmung,** → **psychogene Lähmung.**

läppisches Benehmen puerilism.
This is the term used in psychiatric contexts denoting childish or foolish behavior. Adjective: *puerile. N.B.: puerili***ty** has also a legal connotation: the civil law status of a boy between the ages of 7 and 14, and of a girl between 7 and 12.

Langzeitneuroleptika long-term neuroleptics.
A group of psychopharmaceuticals that have a good antipsychotic effect, little sleep-inducing action, and are consequently very suitable for long-term therapy. → **Breitbandneuroleptika.** → Fig. 3.

Ref.: PÖLDINGER: Compendium of Psychopharmacotherapy, p. 119. Editiones Roche, Basle 1984.

larvierte Depression masked depression.
Psychosomatic symptoms occur in episodes and are associated with a measure of depressive mood. Symptoms such as headache often hide or "mask" actual depression.

latenter Trauminhalt → **Trauminhalt**

Latenzperiode, *Syn.:* **Latenzphase, Latenzzeit** latency; latency stage; latency period.
In psychoanalysis the term covers the phase between the end of the oedipal stage and the onset of puberty, i.e. roughly from the fifth to the twelfth year of life. It is marked by an apparent standstill in psychosexual development (sublimation and repression).

Lebensangst fear for one's life.
This is the general meaning referring to a direct threat to one's life. In the sense in which it is employed by VON UEXKÜLL, however, it comes close to *existential anxiety*. The German term should not be confused with "life fear", which was used by OTTO RANK for the feeling of dread said to be experienced during the process of being born and the consequent urge to return to the safety of the womb.

Lebensdrang élan vital.
This is the term given to the force of vitalism by HENRI BERGSON (1859–1941). Vitalism is the theory that an inorganic force plays an important role in the functions and growth of living matter. The concept was supported by HANS DRIESCH (1867–1941).

Lebensereignis life event (WOLFF).
An unfavorable – or favorable – event in the life of an individual that is of significance in restructuring his life and/or producing illness. *Life-events research* came into being after morbidity studies had shown that episodes of illness occurred in clusters that appeared to be related to environmental changes. RAHE, HOLMES, PAYKEL und others then attempted to quantify the effect of life-changes.

Ref.: CRISP, A. H.: Bereavement. Hexagon 'Roche' 14, No. 1 (1986).
Oxford Textbook of Psychiatry [6], p. 90.

Lebenslüge (ADLER) life lie.
1. Neurotic conviction of the inevitable failure of the life plan (→ **Lebensplan**), possibly with a view to avoiding responsibility. **2.** A false hypothesis underlying the life plan.

Lebensplan (ADLER) life plan.
The plan of an individual to attain ideal or practical goals. This plan determines his style of life and behavior.

Lebenstrieb Eros; life instinct.
The drive opposing the death instinct or Thanatos in FREUD's theory of the instincts. It thus comprises the instinct of self-preservation (→ **Selbsterhaltungstrieb**) and the sexual instinct. → **Trieb.**

Lebensunlust weariness of life.
"Life unpleasure" would be a literal translation, but "unpleasure" has a more specific meaning in psychoanalysis (→ **Unlust**). Alternatives would be *languor* in the sense of *lack of vigor,* and even the more colloquial *being fed up with life.*

Legasthenie → Leseschwäche

Lehranalyse didactic analysis, tuitional analysis, training analysis.
Training in which an analytic candidate undergoes psychoanalysis. He thus not only learns the principles and techniques at first hand, but acquires insight into his own sensitivities and reactions that might result in countertransference (→ **Gegenübertragung**).

Leibbewusstsein somatognosia.
A healthy awareness of one's own body as a functional entity.

leibliches Beeinflussungserlebnis somatic hallucination.
False physical perceptions, e.g. electric currents flowing through the body or the presence of cancer. Frequently encountered in paranoid schizophrenia.

Leidensdruck 1. degree (or level) of suffering. **2.** incentive to get well; motivation to recover.
Unfortunately, neither of these suggestions covers the German meaning entirely. Particularly in the case of neurotics, primary and secondary gains play a role, so that the second alternative would be more appropriate. In order to cover both connotations the term would have to be paraphrased along the following lines: *the degree of suffering motivating recovery.*
3. In some cases the term may refer to the readiness of the patient to seek medical or psychiatric help.

Leim-Schnüffeln glue-sniffing.
A form of substance abuse. The usual ingredient that produces the psychoactive effects is toluene.

Leistung → Fehlleistung, → Hirnleistungsschwäche.

Leistungsgesellschaft meritocracy; performance-oriented society.

Leistungsmotivation achievement motivation (H. MURRAY; D. C. MCCLELLAND).
The need to increase one's performance and overcome difficulties. People with a high degree of achievement motivation usually set themselves higher standards than others, but opinions may differ on this point, particularly with respect to children.

Lernen am Erfolg → operante Konditionierung.

Leseschwäche legasthenia.
Problems with learning to read owing to difficulties in synthesizing individual letters into a word pattern or analyzing a word into its parts. Individuals with this disorder may possess normal intelligence in other fields. *Dyslexia* is similar, but may involve brain lesions.

Letalität(szahl) case fatality rate; fatality rate. The percentage of deaths caused by a disease in relation to the total number of cases of that particular disease. *cf.* **Mortalität.**

Leugnung denial. → **Realitätsleugnung.**

Libido → **Ichlibido,** → **Objektlibido.**

Libidobesetzung libido cathexis.
According to FREUD, the libido can be invested in one's own person (narcissistic) or in an external object. → **Ichlibido,** → **Objektlibido.**

Liebe → **Affenliebe.**

Liebeswahn erotic paranoia; erotic delusion.
A delusional conviction of being loved by another person, usually wealthy or famous. Not to be confused with **Liebeswut** or **Liebestollheit,** which is "erotomania" or "aidoiomania" (preoccupation with sexual activities).

Liebeszwang aphrodisiomania.
An extreme state of mental sexual excitement.

Lösungsmittelschnüffeln volatile chemical inhalation. → **Benzinismus.**

Lüge → **Lebenslüge.**

Lust → **Endlust.**

Lustprinzip pleasure principle.
One of the two most basic principles in human behavior. The organism tends to seek the greatest possible amount of pleasure and to avoid pain. This is modified by the reality principle (→ **Realitätsprinzip**).

Lust-Unlust-Prinzip pleasure-pain principle.
A psychoanalytical principle that people are influenced by opposing desires for pleasurable gratification and for the discharge of tension accumulating as pain or displeasure ("unpleasure") when such gratification is absent.

lustvolles Hergeben voluptuous generosity.

Lykantrophie → **metamorphotischer Wahn.**

M

Machtstreben will to power; strivings for power.
The first expression is the more literal translation of NIETZSCHE's term **Wille zur Macht,** which in his philosophy replaced FREUD's concept of libido as an important driving force. It is often interpreted as an overcompensation for feelings of inferiority.
Ref.: ALEXANDER [1].

Magenausheberung evacuation of the stomach (by pumping).

Magenspülung gastric lavage.

Magersucht emaciation; (pathological) loss of weight.
This may be due to faulty nutrition or disease, e.g. endocrine disorders. The word **Sucht** here is used in its old sense of *'illness'* and has no psychological connotation (as in the term „Wassersucht" = edema). **Magersucht** is a vague word sometimes loosely employed for any extreme loss of weight and sometimes *wrongly* translated as "anorexia nervosa", which would be either → **psychogene Magersucht** or → **Pubertätsmagersucht.** Strictly speaking, "anorexia" means loss of appetite.

Managerkrankheit executive stress.
A condition experienced by some management personnel who carry heavy responsibilities and/or must make important decisions, particularly under hectic circumstances. The stress may manifest itself in such forms as autonomic regulatory disturbances and circulatory disorders.

Mangelsituation → **emotionelle Mangelsituation.**

Manie → **gereizte Manie,** → **Räsoniermanie.**

Manieriertheit mannerism.
The adoption of inappropriate, exaggerated and artificial poses and gestures. Stilted, repetitive forms of expression and behavior. This may extend to speech. It is a feature of catatonic schizophrenia.

manifester Trauminhalt → **Trauminhalt**

maskierte Depression → **larvierte Depression.**

Mechanismus (pl. **Mechanismen**) → **Abwehrmechanismen,** → **angeborene Auslösemechanismen.**

Mehrpersonenanordnungen multiple constellations.
When the family or some other group of persons is involved in the patient's illness or treatment.

Meinung opinion → **Schulmeinungen.**

Melodientaubheit amusia.
Inability to recognize tunes; associated with lesion of the left parietal lobe (in right-handed persons). In English it is also sometimes applied to loss of musical expression, though in German this is more **Melodienstummheit.** *Asonia,* or *tone deafness,* is a form of sensory amusia referring specifically to the inability of being able to distinguish differences in pitch.

Merkfähigkeit registration.
The capacity to add new material to the existing memory store.
Ref.: PETERS [11]; Oxford Book of Psychiatry [6], p. 27.

metamorphotischer Wahn; Lykanthropie lycanthropy, lycomania, zoanthropy.
Delusions of transformation (into an animal).

Metapsychologie metapsychology.
The term has two meanings: **1.** *Beyond psychology* the speculative approach involving the relation of mind to universe. It is sometimes associated with *parapsychology* in this sense.
2. In the Freudian sense it involves different approaches to mental processes: dynamic, structural (→ **strukturelle Einteilung**), topographic (→ **topische Einteilung**), economic, genetic, and adaptive.

Methode → **Jacobsonsche Methode.**

Mikronarkose minimal narcosis.

mimische Ausdrucksphänomene facial expressions (indicative of anxiety etc.).

Minderbegabung mental retardation; mental deficiency; oligophrenia.
The German term is sometimes used as a euphemism for this condition. → **geistige Behinderung.**

Minderwertigkeitsgefühl feelings of inferiority.
According to ADLER, this gives rise to the pattern of reactions known as an *inferiority complex* (→ **Minderwertigkeitskomplex**).

Minderwertigkeitskomplex inferiority complex.
Feelings of insecurity and inadequacy stemming from childhood dependence. It may cause some individuals to strive for greater achievement as compensation, while others with personality disorders will tend either to overcompensate (aggression) or to withdraw from all competitive activities.

Missbrauch (von Drogen, Medikamenten) → **Arzneimittelmissbrauch.**

Misshandlungssyndrom → **Kindsmisshandlung.**

Mitbewusstes (M. PRINCE) → **Vorbewusstes.**

Mitgehen mitgehen.
Moving a limb in response to slight pressure, despite being told to resist it. A feature of the schizophrenic defect state.
Ref.: Oxford Textbook of Psychiatry [6], p. 233.

Mortalität mortality.
The percentage of deaths over a specific period of time for the whole population or a specified part of it (e.g. infants). This definition concurs with the accepted German meaning, but *death rate,* which is usually synonymous with mortality, has been defined as the ratio of deaths in a specified area to the total population, usually expressed as the number of deaths per 1,000 or 10,000 etc. of the population. *cf.* **Letalität.**

Motilitätspsychose motility psychosis.
Striking changes in psychomotor activity, from total lack of movement to overactivity. The condition represents one of the cycloid psychoses. → **Angst-Glücks-Psychose.**
Ref.: PETERS [11]; Oxford Textbook of Psychiatry [6], p. 243.

Motivation → **Leistungsmotivation.**

motorische Einstellung motor set.
A predisposition to exert efforts similar to those associated with past tasks.
Ref.: NEEL: [10a] p. 28; [10b], S. 51.

Mündigkeit → **Ehefähigkeit.**

mussitierendes Delirium (Delirium mussitans) muttering delirium.
A type of delirium in which the patient mutters and repeats to himself words that are largely incomprehensible. Speech is slurred

and accompanied by trembling. The condition is generally associated with alcoholism.

Mutterersatz mother surrogate, mother substitute, mother figure.
The first term is preferable. The general meaning is a person who takes over the basic duties and functions of a real mother. However, in psychoanalysis it refers to a person on whom a patient projects feelings or attitudes originally held toward a real mother. The projection itself is an unconscious process.

N

Nachhallpsychose flashback psychosis.
While some authors would object to the world "psychosis" in this sense, *flashback* is a recognized event: the recurrence of psychedelic experience after a drug-free period. *Flashback hallucinosis* is most common after taking LSD, and may occur a considerable period after the drug was last ingested.
Ref.: PETERS [11]; Longman; [7]; Oxford Textbook of Psychiatry [6], p. 453.

Nachreifung delay in development; developmental delay.
In a psychiatric context it will generally be understood that the term refers to *delay in emotional and intellectual development,* but otherwise these words may be added for extra clarity. *ICD-9* lists "Specific Delays in Development" and DSM-III "Specific Development Disorders".
Ref.: Oxford Textbook of Psychiatry [6], p. 663.

Nachtangst sleep-terror disorder; pavor nocturnus; night terror.
Sudden awakening with both emotional and physical symptoms of intense fear: panic, screaming, sweating, dilated pupils, and rapid heartbeat.

Nachtesser night-eater.
The original term was English (U.S.), and is applied to a person who is afflicted by excessive hunger after nightfall. Sleep is consequently troubled and there is reduced appetite on the morning after.

Nachtesser-Syndrom night-eating syndrome.

Nachtklinik → psychiatrische Nachtklinik.

Nahrungsverweigerung apastia.
Abstention from food, either as a neurologic or psychiatric symptom (e.g. in anorexia nervosa). In a more general sense, however, the German expression may be translated simply as *refusal to eat,* particularly in the case of children, or, more formally, *abstinence from food.*

Neid → Penisneid.

Neuroleptika neuroleptics.
Non-barbiturate sedatives with an "antipsychotic effect". Sometimes called *major tranquilizers.* → **Tranquilizer,** → **Basisneuroleptika,** → **Langzeitneuroleptika.**

Neurose → vegetative Neurose, → Abstiegsneurose, → Begehrensneurose, → Berufsneurose, → Beschäftigungsneurose, → Erwartungsneurose, → Kernneurose, → Kriegsneurose, → Organneurose, → Schicksalsneurose, → Unfallneurose, → Zwangsneurose (→ Tab. 1).

Neurosenwahl choice of neurosis. → **Symptomenwahl.**

neurotische Angst neurotic anxiety.
This is difficult to distinguish from moral anxiety, but it belongs to the pathological sphere even if it is a product of conflicts in early childhood. It stems from real conflicts that have been repressed instead of solved.

neurotische Stumpfheit "neurotic obtuseness".
A term relating to patients with habitual headache, which is thought to be the result of intellectual inhibition and negativism.

Nichtbefolgen der ärztlichen Behandlungsmassnahmen noncompliance (with medical treatment).

The converse, "compliance" has now been widely adopted by German writers.

Niveau level, standard. → **Anspruchsniveau.**

Noradrenalin norepinephrine (U.S.), noradrenaline (U.K.).

One of the catecholamines and a neurohormonal transmitter of the postganglionic nerves. In the brain it is probably concerned with mechanisms underlying mood and learning reactions.

Nullbefund no abnormal finding. → **o. B.**

O

o. B. (ohne Befund, ohne Besonderheiten) no abnormal finding. → **Nullbefund**

Objektlibido object libido.
The part of the libido invested in one or more objects of the external world. *Object cathexis* is the concentration or investment of psychic energy in any objects outside the self. *cf.* **Ichlibido.**

Objektverlust object loss.
Loss of a person or impending loss of affection. The term may be extended to include loss of an occupation that meant much to the patient.

Offenbarungswahn religious delusion.
This is sometimes considered as a variation of *grandiose delusion* when the patient believes himself to be a prophet destined to advise on great issues. In an extreme form the patient is convinced he is the Messiah, can save humankind, or may even go so far as to commit rape in order to beget Jesus. The more literal translation *delusions of revelation* has very limited currency.

Oknophil ocnophile.
A type of person who prefers dependence and does not like to take any risk. The entire life strategy of such individuals is centered on being protected. *cf.* **Philobat.** Both terms were coined by M. BALINT.

operante Interventionsverfahren behavior modification. → **operante Konditionierung.**

operante Konditionierung operant conditioning.
The original term was English (SKINNER). The technique consists of giving rewards or "punishment" with respect to the desired behavioral changes. Sometimes employed in treating anorexia nervosa, where the patient is rewarded when a weight gain has been achieved or the reward withheld when a certain weight has not been maintained.

operatives Denken pensée opératoire.
The term stems from MARTY and M'UZAN and refers to the inability to fantasize freely. Patients with this condition are less able to relate dreams, and when they can, the content is usually poor and stereotyped without any symbolic meaning. This is part of the picture of alexithymia (→ **Alexithymic**), a later concept.

oraler Charakter oral character.
Personality traits derived from the oral stage of development. If an individual has gained adequate attention from the mother during the oral-sucking phase, he develops an *oral-receptive* (**oral empfangender**) *character* marked by friendliness, optimism, generosity, and dependence on others. If not, he develops an *oral-aggressive character* marked by hostile, envious, and overcompetitive tendencies.

orales Beißstadium oral-biting period (stage).
In psychoanalysis the second stage of the oral period of psychosexual development.

orales Saugstadium oral-sucking stage; oral eroticism phase.
In psychoanalysis the first phase of psychosexual development.
Ref.: NEEL [10]; Longman [7].

Organe der prärationalen Psyche archetypes.
The German term given was used by JUNG in

1935 to refer to his *archetypes,* structural components of the mind derived from man's accumulated experience.

Ref.: Frey-Rohn, L.: Von Freud zu Jung, S. 135. Daimon, Zürich 1969.

Organminderwertigkeit organ inferiority.

Adler's term for organic defects of any kind, including imaginary, that result in feelings of inferiority and attempts to compensate.

Organneurose organ neurosis.

A functional disorder incurring a physiological change. Psychological factors may affect a physical condition. *cf.* **Organpsychose.**

Organpsychose organ psychosis (by analogy with **Organneurose** organ neurosis).

Denotes a condition in which a physiological change occurs in any organ as a result of psychotic features. It should not be confused with "organ**ic** psychosis" in English, which is "organic brain syndrome" (→ **Psychosyndrom**).

Organsprache organ language; hypochondriac language.

Physical expressions of emotional conflicts, for which the symptoms have symbolic significance. The term is sometimes used interchangeably with *body language,* but the infrequently used Adlerian expression *organ jargon* is something rather different: physical disturbances, such as constipation, that are said to be the neurotic expression of a masculine protest against feminine symptoms of weakness.

Ref.: Longman [7].

Orientierung → örtliche Orientierung, → räumliche Orientierung.

orthodoxer Schlaf orthodox sleep, non-REM sleep, slow-wave sleep.

Non-REM sleep (now the more prevalent term) is divided into four stages: In the first the EEG is akin to the waking EEG. Stage two shows a new feature of sleep spindles, which give way to slow waves, which in turn increasingly dominate the picture as stage four is reached. *cf.* **paradoxer Schlaf.**

örtliche Orientierung orientation of place.

The ability to determine and recognize one's present location, e.g. that one is in hospital or in an old people's home. *cf.* **räumliche Orientierung.**

P

Paartherapie marriage therapy, marital therapy, couples therapy.
Treatment aimed at altering the psychodynamics and behavior of the partners to improve marital relationships. Grievances may be aired, but sometimes analytic techniques are used to reveal the source of defensive or aggressive attitudes.

Pädagogik → Heilpädagogik.

paradoxer Schlaf paradoxical sleep, REM sleep.
One of the major classes of sleep. The latter term appears to be replacing the former both in English and German (**REM-Schlaf**). In this type of sleep an individual cannot easily be awakened, although it would seem to be light sleep according to the EEG. It is also the sleep in which dreams occur. REM (rapid eye movement) sleep is the fifth stage in the new classification, the other four being non-rapid eye movement sleep (NREM). *cf.* **orthodoxer Schlaf.**

Paralyse → jugendliche Paralyse.

Partialtrieb component instinct; part-instinct; partial instinct.
A psychoanalytic term for an instinct connected with a particular zone (e.g. oral or anal) that continues to provide gratification when such zones become subordinated to genital areas.
Ref.: Longman [7].

passagerer Tic transient-tic disorder *(DSM-III)*.
Involuntary and inappropriate twitches usually occurring up to adolescence. The duration of the disorder is generally greater than one month but less than a year.
Ref.: Longman [7].

pathologischer Rausch, *Syn.:* **alkoholischer Dämmerzustand** alcohol idiosyncratic intoxication *(DSM-III)*.
Radical change in behavior after imbibing even moderate amounts of alcohol. Frequent symptoms are aggressivity, sometimes violence (although the individual may normally be of a mild, retiring disposition) and amnesia. There are various opinions as to the causes, as there are about the terminology. Also called *mania a potu, pathological intoxication.*

Penisneid penis envy, phallus envy.
The desire of the female to possess a male genital organ.

per explorationem by examination.

Perfektionismus → Vollkommenheitswahn.

persistierende Dyskinesien → dyskinetische Spätsyndrome.

Person → Bezugsperson.

persönliches Unbewusstes personal unconscious.
That part of the unconscious containing the components of personal experience. → Fig. 2.

Persönlichkeit → Entkernung der Persönlichkeit, → hypersensitive Persönlichkeitsstörung, → prämorbide Persönlichkeit, → Primärpersönlichkeit, → psychopathische Persönlichkeit, → Risikopersönlichkeit.

Persönlichkeitsabbau → Hirnleistungsschwäche.

Persönlichkeitsbild 1. personality profile.
A description of personal attributes and traits

that distinguish one personality from another. There is often a "personality profile" common to patients suspectible to a given disorder.

2. Dimensions of personality (in EYSENCK's sense). → Fig. 5.

Ref.: TILLEARD-COLE, R. R.: Aspects of Personality for Medical Practice. Hexagon 'Roche' 6, No. 4 (1978).

Persönlichkeitsspaltung dual personality.
A dissociative disorder in which the original personality is usually unaware of the other personality that is, according to M. PRINCE, "split-off and independently acting". When several subpersonalities are involved one speaks of *multiple personality*. The lay term "split personality", often confused with schizophrenia, should be avoided.

Pfropfschizophrenie (not translated). Of historical interest only, the term referred to a form of schizophrenia that was thought to be superimposed onto mental retardation.

Phantasien → Urphantasien.

Philobat philobate.
A venturesome person who accepts risks and dislikes dependence, as opposed to the ocnophile (→ **Oknophil**). Both terms were coined by M. BALINT.

Phobien phobias. → Appendix.

physiologisches Bedürfnis → primäres Bedürfnis.

Polaritätsprofil semantic differential (OSGOOD).
A graphical method of measuring the connotation of a concept for an individual by rating it on a seven-point scale with reference to pairs of opposites, e.g. on the left may be the words "weak", "cold" etc. and on the right "strong", "hot" etc., these being separated by seven columns.
Ref.: PETERS [11]; Longman [7].

Pollution nocturnal emission.
Involuntary ejaculation occurring during a dream, hence the popular term *wet dream*. One meaning of the English word "pollution" corresponds to this, but its use is infrequent in this sense, and it is usually employed as an equivalent to the German **Verschmutzung** or **Umweltverschmutzung** (pollution of the environment).

Polyarthritis, primär chronische
Rheumatoid arthritis is usually meant, but the term may cover other polyarthritic conditions.

Polypragmasie polypharmacy.
The use of several drugs in treating the same patient. This is necessary in special cases but it may lead to "polydrug addiction" (dependence on a variety of drugs).

positive Erinnerungsfälschung pseudomemory; (formerly: pseudomnesia).
A fictitious "recall" of events that exist only in the imagination. → **Erinnerungsfälschung.**

Potenzstörung sexual dysfunction.
An overall term covering general inability to complete the sex act. It includes premature and retrograde ejaculation, coitus without ejaculation, failure to maintain erection, but also priapism.
Sexual dysfunction in women would include frigidity, anorgasmia, vaginismus, and dyspareunia.
Ref.: PETERS [11]; Longman [7].

Prädelirium tremens subdelirious state; subdelirium.
The precursor of a full delirium, before the disorientation stage.

prägende Einflüsse shaping influences.
An example would be loss of a parent during childhood or puberty. In this instance "shaping" is employed in a different sense than in → **Verhaltensformung.**

Ref.: CRISP, A. H.: Bereavement. Hexagon Roche 14/1 (1986) 14.

Prägnanzregel principle of Prägnanz.
A concept of gestalt psychology claiming that perceptual experiences acquire complete, meaningful forms when evaluated in the mind. Examples are filling out gaps in a story to make it complete and making words out of individual letters. (**Prägnanz** [literally] = terseness, precision).

Prägung imprinting.
In the wider sense the term may refer to any lasting influence of educational and social environment. In the narrower sense it is a primitive, rapid, but stable learning pattern in the critical, early life of a social animal. It involves identification with its own species or even with a surrogate in order to form family relations.

prämorbide Persönlichkeit premorbid personality.
Previous personality defects predisposing to another mental disorder.

Präsentiersymptom "proposed symptom".
M. BALINT's contention was that the patient may seek out a symptom which brings him to the doctor but which has little relevance to his underlying illness. One cannot therefore speak of a "presenting symptom" in the medical sense. When, however, such a patient comes from a psychologically sick family unit he may himself be termed a "presenting symptom" of the family illness.

Prävalenz → Häufigkeitsquotient.

Primärerlebnis → schizophrenes Primärerlebnis.

primäres Bedürfnis primary need.
The need to satisfy a physiological need, e.g. breathing, eating, sleeping, etc. Primary need is unlearned and stems from biological processes. → **sekundäres Bedürfnis** (secondary need).

Primärpersönlichkeit premorbid personality.
A patient's personality prior to onset of disease. It may constitute a predisposing factor to the type of illness or reaction.

Primärprozess primary process.
Unconscious mental activity with uninhibited, instinctual discharge. → **Es** *(id)*. Such processes give rise to "primary process thinking". *cf.* → **Sekundärprozess.** Primary processes ignore the restrictions imposed by one's social milieu or by the external world in general. In other words, such processes are more emotional than rational, their expression pictorial rather than verbal.

Primärwahn autochthonous delusion; primary delusion.
A delusion appearing "of itself" for no apparent reason. It is more a delusional idea or conviction than a perception or hallucination.

primitive Affektreaktion isolated explosive disorder; catathymic crisis.
An impulse control disorder involving a single, violent outburst that is not mediated by the rational personality. The act is out of all proportion to the circumstances and unwarranted. In popular terms it is often described as *going berserk,* but this precise disorder may end in suicide. → **Kurzschlusshandlung.**

Prinzip → Lustprinzip, → Lust-Unlust-Prinzip, → Realitätsprinzip.

Proskinesie repeated and forced grasping.
The patient may grasp an outstretched hand despite instructions to the contrary. Often associated with → **Mitgehen** in catatonic schizophrenia.

Protest → Pubertätsprotest.

Prozess → **Primärprozess,** → **Sekundärprozess.**

Prozess-Schizophrenie process schizophrenia.
A debatable term referring to early, chronic forms of the disease that are thought to be endogenous or constitutional in origin. The patients are extremely withdrawn and indulge in fantasies. *Process psychosis* is similar, but terminates in permanent dementia. → **ausgebrannt.**

Prüfung test, examination. → **Realitätsprüfung.**

Pseudologia phantastica
The Latin term is used in both languages but the spelling *pseudologia fantastica* will be found in English. Despite the possible nuance existing between "phantasy" and "fantasy" in English (→ **Urphantasien**) this is a dubious practice if the expression is supposed to be Latin. The term relates to a syndrome in which an individual concocts fantastic lies in order to impress others.

Psyche → **Organe der prärationalen Psyche,** → Fig. 2.

psychiatrische Begutachtung expert witness testimony.
The statement of a person qualified to act as consultant in legal procedures connected with forensic psychiatry.

psychiatrische Nachtklinik night hospital.
Psychiatric care is afforded patients in the evening and during the night, while they spend the daytime in the general community.
Ref.: PETERS [11]; Longman [7].

psychischer Apparat psychic apparatus; mental apparatus.
FREUD's expression describing a basic model for psychic processes. It constitutes an overall term for the various levels of consciousness and their relationship to the id, ego, and superego.

psychischer Befund mental status (U.S.); mental state (U.K.).
The psychological condition of a patient at the time of a mental (state) examination with respect to many factors, including general intelligence, emotional state, motor activity, sensory awareness, and judgment.

psychischer Konflikt intrapsychic conflict.
The clash of two conflicting desires, motivations or ambitions. → **innerseelischer Konflikt.**

psychogalvanischer Reflex (PGR) galvanic skin response (GSR); psychogalvanic reflex (PGR).
A change in electrical resistance of the skin as a response to stimuli. It is produced by sweat gland activity.

psychogene Blindheit *Syn.:* **funktionelle Blindheit, hysterische Blindheit, pithiatische Blindheit** hysterical blindness; hysterical amaurosis.
A hysterical conversion symptom representing an unconscious attempt to "close the eyes" to a threatening or guilt-laden situation. The patient's sight is totally or partially impaired, yet the pupils continue to react to light.

psychogene Lähmung hysterical paralysis; conversion paralysis.
Paralysis without any organic cause. A conversion symptom.

psychogene Magersucht anorexia nervosa. → **Magersucht.**

psychogene psychotische Episode episodic behavior disorder.
Brief periods of behavior that are atypical of the individual and may be impulsive, possibly ending in violence or suicide.

psychogener Tod psychogenic death.
The German expression is mostly used to mean *voodoo death.* This is culture-specific, the victim being literally "frightened to death" (CANNON) by the ceremony of the medicine man who condemns him.

psychogenes Weglaufen psychogenic fugue *(DSM-III);* fugue.
Running away from home or the accustomed environment and assuming a fresh identity. The first "life" is usually forgotten, but can be recalled spontaneously or by treatment. In German, the term → **Fugue** is limited to children wandering aimlessly away from home, and is synonymous with → **Poriomanie,** which is not quite the same as the English term poriomania.
→ **Fortlaufen.**

Psychologie → analytische Psychologie, → Entwicklungspsychologie, → Gestaltpsychologie, → komplexe Psychologie, → Metapsychologie, → Tiefenpsychologie.

Psycholytika psycholytics.
Hallucinogenic agents; drugs producing a model psychosis, which can also be used to support psychotherapy.

Psychomotorik psychomotility.
Movements shaped by psychic processes. This includes characteristic gaits, handwriting, tics, and speech. Adjective: **psychomotorisch** psychomotor.

psychomotorischer Anfall **1.** psychomotor epilepsy; temporal lobe epilepsy.
An attack comprising various forms of paramnesia, repetitive movements including swallowing and chewing, and vague hallucinations. The patient usually appears to be in a dreamy state, which may resemble a trance.
2. dreamy state.
An altered state of consciousness which includes brief olfactory, visual, and auditory hallucinations but no convulsions.
The German terms **psychomotorischer Anfall** and → **Dämmerattacke** are often synonymous, which is unfortunate considering the distinctions made by the two English terms.

psychomotorisch dämpfend psychomotor sedative.
A term describing the properties of a class of antidepressants.

psychopathische Persönlichkeit psychopathic personality.
The *Oxford Textbook of Psychiatry* [6] avoids the term, employing *personality disorder* in the wider sense, and *antisocial personality* in the narrower sense.

psychosexuelle Entwicklungsstadien psychosexual levels (of development).

Psychose → Angst-Glücks-P., → Einheitspsychose, → Fieberpsychose, → Freiheitspsychose, → funktionelle Psychose, → Funktionspsychose, → Gefängnispsychose, → Haftpsychose, → Intoxikationspsychose, → Kinderpsychose, → Mortalitätspsychose, → Nachhallpsychose, → Organpsychose, → Randpsychose, → symbiontische Psychose, → symbiotische Psychose.

Psychosomatik psychosomatic medicine.
This English term is preferable to "psychosomatics", and even in German the tendency is to favor **psychosomatische Medizin.** It is then clear that one is referring to an approach that takes into account both the organic and psychological factors of disease, and not a separate discipline.

psychosomatisch
The long accepted translation *psychosomatic* has recently come under fire from some quarters, the contention being that the term suggests a mind-body dualism. The expression *psychophysiologic* has been proposed, but does not this suggest a 'mind-physiologic' dualism? The *WHO Glossary of Mental Disorders*

(1981) lists both terms as NOS (not otherwise stated) under a main classification "physiological malfunction arising from mental factors".
Moreover, the term psychophysiologic would come into conflict with the German term **psychophysiologisch** as defined in earlier classifications by ENGEL and by HEIM, where **psychophysiologische Störungen** were called psychosomatic disorders "in the wider sense" as distinguished from those "in the narrower sense".
Until general agreement has been reached, it would thus seem advisable to continue using the term *psychosomatic.*

psychosomatische Krankheit psychosomatic disease (or illness).
The term is used loosely in practice, but it would be well to reserve it for cases where organic change has taken place. → **psychosomatische Störung.**

psychosomatisches Kreuz
Although **Kreuz** can sometimes be translated as *"the small of the back"* it refers obliquely to the *sacrum* **(Kreuzbein),** this being the region where frequently injury is sustained when, for example, a person slips on his back. In this context, however, it also refers to "the cross one has to bear". The term is thus a play on words for which it is difficult to find an English equivalent, and is best paraphrased.

psychosomatische Störung psychosomatic disturbance (or disorder).
The word *disorder* in particular is used very loosely, but it may prove advisable to restrict both *disturbance* and *disorder* to describe conditions in which there was originally no organic change, but a functional disorder in which a physiological change eventually occurs. The term may thus often be replaced by *organ neurosis.*

psychosomatisches Training psychosomatic training.
A combination of exercises centered around breathing, which may in individual cases be supplemented by massage aimed at relaxation. Originated by B. LUBAN-PLOZZA and W. PÖLDINGER.

Psychosyndrom; hirnorganisches Psychosyndrom organic brain syndrome, organic psychosis.
Mental disorders caused by or associated with impairment of brain tissue function. The second term listed is confusing, since such disorders may be psychotic or nonpsychotic. It may, moreover, be confused with the newly improvised term "organ psychosis" (→ **Organpsychose**) which is something quite different from *organ***ic** *psychosis.*

Psychotherapie → aufdeckende Psychotherapie, → klientenzentrierte Psychotherapie, → unterstützende Psychotherapie, → zudeckende Psychotherapie.

psychotische Angst psychotic anxiety.
This occurs in endogenous depression, schizophrenia or organic psychoses.

psychovegetativ → vegetativ.

Pubertätsmagersucht anorexia nervosa. → **Magersucht.**

Pubertätsprotest → Trotzverhalten.

Punkte → hysterische Punkte.

Q

Quälsucht sadism.
Regarded by some authorities as a sexual deviation, by others as a perversion, in which gratification is obtained by inflicting pain or humiliation; but the practice may be extended beyond the sexual partner to, for example, animals.

quantifizierbar able to be measured or quantitated.
Examples: **quantifizierbares Farbwahlverhalten** color-choice behavior that can be measured (or quantitated). **Unquantifizierbar** not subject to being quantitated.

Quartalsäufer dipsomaniac.
A periodic or *binge drinker*. Bouts of heavy drinking may be interspersed with dry periods as in epsilon alcoholism. **Quartalsaufen** dipsomania.

Querulantenwahn litigious paranoia, paranoia querulans, paranoid litigious state, querulous paranoia.
The first term is more common, since the patient often has a tendency to go to law, usually for imaginary causes, but he is also inclined to quarrel in addition to claiming persecution. There is thus some overlap with "delusion of persecution" (→ **Verfolgungswahn**).

Quotient → **Gefahrenquotient,** → **Häufigkeitsquotient,** → **Risikoquotient.**

R

Randbewusstsein marginal consciousness; fringe of consciousness.
Conscious content that is not the direct focus of attention.

Randpsychosen cycloid marginal psychoses.
Functional psychoses that are neither typically schizophrenic nor manic-depressive.
Ref.: Oxford Textbook of Psychiatry [6], p. 243.

Räsoniermanie reasoning mania.
Originally *folie raisonnante* described by SERIEUX and CAPGRAS. The patient persistently reasons about some problem or topic which he knows is absurd or which does not really concern or interest him.
Ref.: BRILL [2].

räumliche Orientierung spatial orientation.
The ability to find one's way about one's own dwelling or familiar surroundings. *cf.* **örtliche Orientierung.**

Rausch drunkenness; intoxication.
Originally: *mild drunkenness; euphoriant effect,* e.g. with amphetamines. **Der grosse Rausch** (in drug taking) high (slang). **berauscht:** lit up (slang).
→ **pathologischer Rausch.**
Ref.: Lebende Sprachen 4, Juli/August 1970; Oxford Textbook of Psychiatry [6], p. 451.

Rauschesser binge eater.
A person who is suddenly overcome by a voracious appetite and consumes enormous quantities of food before he is satisfied. The recurrent disorder is known as the *binge-eating syndrome.*

Rauschinhalt (LEUNER)
Material elicited under the influence of psycholytic therapy (now largely obsolete).

Räuspertic laryngeal tic.
A throat-clearing tic. Noisy expulsion of air through the glottis. Also, *hawking,* uttering a sound as if trying to clear the throat of phlegm.

Reaktionsbildung reaction formation.
Development of a behavior pattern in which repressed impulses are denied by diametrically opposed action. *Example:* a mother may be overindulgent to a child she rejects or even hates. This is one of the defense mechanisms (→ **Abwehrmechanismen**).

reaktives Bedürfnis → **sekundäres Bedürfnis.**

Realangst real anxiety.
Anxiety caused by true dangers posed by the external world of reality. It thus constitutes a valuable signal of alarm.

Realitätskontrolle control imposed by reality.

Realitätsleugnung scotomization.
Turning a "blind eye" to external facts. A form of defense mechanism.

Realitätsprinzip reality principle.
Foregoing immediate gratification or postponing it until a more opportune moment owing to external pressures, e.g. the work at hand. It also comes into play when a patient is willing to undergo a certain amount of pain for therapeutic reasons. In other words, it modifies the pleasure principle (→ **Lustprinzip**).

Realitätsprüfung reality testing.
In the psychoanalytical sense this means the objective evaluation by an individual of im-

pressions given by the senses, enabling him or her to distinguish between fantasy and reality. Impairment of this faculty is a major sign of psychosis.

Redekur talking cure.
Sometimes a pejorative term suggesting that psychoanalysis consists mainly of talking about problems and events. It was first employed by "Anna O." in referring to BREUER's cathartic method. → **Breuer-Verfahren.**

Reflex → bedingter Reflex, → psychogalvanischer Reflex, → saltatorischer Reflex, → Totstellreflex, → unbedingter Reflex.

Regel 1. rule. → **Abstinenzregel.**
2. menstrual period. *Syn.* **Regelblutung, „die Tage“** (colloquial).

regredieren to regress.
In the psychoanalytical sense, to revert to earlier, immature, and well-established habits.

Regression regression.
Return to an earlier (infantile) behavior pattern in psychic development, usually under stress or illness. This is the psychoanalytic meaning, which was taken over from the Darwinian concept of regression in the evolutionary phases of certain species. *cf.* **Fixierung.**

Reim → Schüttelreim.

Reizgeneralisierung stimulus generalization.
The tendency for a conditioned response to be elicited by stimuli similar to the conditioned stimulus. *Example:* a child who almost drowns in the bathtub may develop a fear of boating or swimming in later life.

Reizüberflutung flooding.
A radical technique in behavior therapy in which the patient is exposed repeatedly to the fear-producing situation. *Example:* Goethe is said to have cured himself of vertigo by repeated visits to the spire of Strasbourg cathedral. The technique comes under the general heading of *exposure treatments. Implosion* is similar, using an exaggerated conception of the fear. Both methods tend to be replaced by *desensitization. cf.* **Angsthierarchie.**

Reproduktionsfähigkeit 1. recall (→ **Abruf**). **2.** reproduction.
In the memory sense, this may also be defined as a revival of what has previously been learned, but it is sometimes used in the sense that a task is repeated in the manner in which it was learned originally. The biological connotation should be clear from the context. *N.B.* The German should not be confused with *reproductive facilitation,* which refers to an improvement in reproducing a response acquired by learning.

Rhythmus rhythm, cycle. → **Schlaf-Wach-Rhythmus.**

Risikopersönlichkeit personality at risk.

Risikoquotient risk of drug dependence; dependence risk factor.
This may refer to the drug used (heroin would constitute a high-dependence risk factor). The German term is sometimes used interchangeably with → **Gefahrenquotient.**
Ref.: MARKS, J.: The Benzodiazepines, p. 80. MTP Press, Lancaster 1978.

Rollenwechsel role shift.
Strictly speaking, the exchange in roles between two partners. It is, however, extended to the adoption by one member of a group of the characteristic behavior of another, e.g. the loss of the father in the family unit may vacate a role that can be taken up by the son.
Ref.: Longman [7]; CRISP, A. H.: Bereavement. Hexagon 'Roche' 14/1 (1986) 13.

Rückbildungsalter age of physical and psychological deterioration; involution.
The second term is often used in connection with the menopause. The old term "involutional melancholy" has now been replaced by *involutional psychotic reaction.*

Rückschau retrospection.
A review of one's own past experience.

Rücktransport (Psychopharmaka)retransport.

Rückzug withdrawal (in the sense of retreat).
Withdrawal reaction would in many cases be more specific when one speaks of a defensive reaction such as withdrawal from social contact or menacing situations. The term is then differentiated from *withdrawal symptoms* (→ **Entziehungserscheinungen**).

Rührseligkeit oversensitiveness to emotional stimuli; emotional overreaction.
The quality of being easily moved (to tears), e.g. by some tragic event in the distant past.

S

saltatorischer Reflex → **Bambergersche Krankheit.**

Säufer → **Quartalsäufer.**

schabende Schmerzen gnawing pains.

Schatten shadow; shadow self.
One of JUNG's archetypes, which he regards as a moral problem that challenges the ego personality. It constitutes instincts inherited mainly from sexual and aggressive components that are repressed into the personal unconscious → **persönliches Unterbewusstsein,** where they may form "complexes".
Ref.: The Portable Jung [3], p. 145.

Schätzskala rating scale.
A scale used to assess characteristics and abilities of a given individual.

Scheinschwangerschaft → **eingebildete Schwangerschaft.**

Schicksalsanalyse (SZONDI) fate analysis.
A type of depth therapy attempting to discover the "plan" behind the patient's life. This is held to be determined by genetic factors stemming from the "familial unconscious". → **familiäres Unbewusstes**; → Fig. 2.

Schicksalsneurose destiny neurosis; fate neurosis.
The patient appears to be plagued by repeated quirks of fate, for which, according to psychoanalysis, he is himself to blame: he arranges his life in such a manner that they are bound to recur.

Schiefhals torticollis; wryneck.
A disorder of movement. One-sided twisting of the neck may be psychogenic or neurologic in origin, spasmodic or continuous in nature.

schizophrenes Primärerlebnis delusional perception.
A schizophrenic patient's new interpretation of his environment during the initial stages of the disease, in that fresh significance may be attached to a percept without reason. The arrangement of certain familiar objects, or their changed order, may be interpreted, for example, as having a divine or supernatural significance that is of personal concern. → **Wahnstimmung.**

Schizophrenie → **Pfropfschizophrenie,** → **Prozess-Schizophrenie**

Schlaf → **Ammenschlaf-Phänomen,** → **Einschlafdenken,** → **Einschlafstörungen,** → **Einschlafzeremoniell,** → **orthodoxer Schlaf,** → **paradoxer Schlaf.**

Schlafentzugsbehandlung sleep deprivation (treatment).
It has been suggested that certain depressive patients can be helped (e.g. suicidal tendencies prevented) by depriving them of sleep for, say, 24 hours. At present subject to further study.
Ref.: PETERS [11]; Oxford Textbook of Psychiatry [6], p. 219.

Schlaf-Wach-Rhythmus sleep-wake cycle.
Alternating periods of sleep and wakefulness controlled by the brain. *A disruption of the sleep-wake cycle* **(Schlaf-Wach-Störung)** may arise due to "jet lag", night shifts, sleep inversion, or drugs.

Schlafzeremoniell → **Einschlafzeremoniell.**

Schlüsselerlebnis (KRETSCHMER) key event (literal translation); a personality-specific, critical event.
An intensive experience that precipitates an abnormal emotional state. Such an event may only be critical in emotional development for a certain type of personality. In some cases it may be a *life event* (→ **Lebensereignis**), but this is of more significance to the life structure of the individual than to a given personality structure.
The second English term suggested is more of a definition, and there is a tendency on the part of British and American authors to use more specific expressions where appropriate. *Examples:* 1. A *precipitating event* could induce what KRETSCHMER called "sensitive delusions of reference" (**der sensitive Beziehungswahn**). 2. When sensitive people are faced with a deeply *humiliating experience* they develop suspicious ideas. 3. a non-specific vulnerability to *stressful events*.
Ref.: English examples abstracted from the Oxford Textbook of Psychiatry [6], pp. 275, 113, 250.

Schmerz(en) pain(s). → **schabende Schmerzen,** → **Spannungskopfschmerzen.**

Schmerzanfälligkeit-Syndrom pain-prone syndrome.
This term overlaps a good deal with the "depression-pain syndrome" (→ **Depressions-Schmerz-Syndrom**), but also covers some atypical cases characterized by chronic pain where depression is often overlooked. This comes under the main heading of "masked depression" (→ **larvierte Depression**).

Schmerzasymbolie pain asymbolia.
The perception of a painful stimulus without recognizing it as painful.

Schmerzgeilheit (slang) → **Algolagnie.**

Schock → **Affektschock,** → **Granatschock.**

Schreckblitz auditory-visual synesthesia.
A form of crossed perception in which loud noises may be experienced visually, e.g. as bright spots or vague patches, before the eyes.

Schuld debt; fault. → **Traumschuld.**

Schulmeinungen pedantic notions.

Schulschwierigkeiten academic problems (DSM-III); academic-underachievement disorder.
Failing to "move up" at school or make the grade at university despite adequate intelligence and absence of any specific mental or developmental disturbance. The expressions *school problems* and *difficulties at school* may be simpler, but they may also cover problems arising with schoolmates or fellow students.

Schüttelreim
Example: „Es soll der Mosel Sonnenwein uns Inbegriff der Wonnen sein".
The German expression is attributed to ANTON KIPPENBERG (1874–1950). The English equivalent is *spoonerism,* from the clergyman SPOONER (1844–1930), who was known to make mistakes in transposing initial sounds. *English examples:* "Stand back and let the parson cough!" (instead of "stand back and let the coffin pass!"). "This way lady, I will sew you into a sheet" ("... I will show you into a seat").

Schwäche → **Hirnleistungsschwäche,** → **Leseschwäche.**

Schwachsinn feeblemindedness; mental retardation; oligophrenia. → **Altersschwachsinn.**

Schwangerschaft pregnancy. → **eingebildete Schwangerschaft,** → **Scheinschwangerschaft.**

Schweigepflicht confidentiality.
The ethical principle that physicians and

other therapists should not divulge information obtained from the patient. In some countries this extends to other medical personnel, dentists and pharmacists, while other states do not recognize the principle at all if such information is required for legal proceedings.
Ref.: Brit. med. J. 285 (1982) 1655.

Schweiss sweat, perspiration. → **Angstschweiss.**

Schwerbesinnlichkeit poverty of thought.
A condition in which the patient has few thoughts; even these lack in variety and richness and appear to move slowly through the mind.
Ref.: Oxford Textbook of Psychiatry [6], p. 9.

Schwierigkeit → **Schulschwierigkeiten.**

Seele mind, soul, psyche.
There has been controversy, but *mind* is the usual translation in the field covered by this book.
Ref.: HARE, E.: Freud, thou art translated. Brit. med. J. 287 (1983) 1293–1294.
The adjective **seelisch** is usually rendered by *mental* and sometimes *emotional,* e.g. **seelische Leere** emotional vacuum, **abnorme seelische Reaktion** abnormal emotional reaction (a vague term, usually a synonym for neurosis).

Seelsorge → **Telefonseelsorge.**

sekundäres Bedürfnis secondary need.
A need acquired by learning to satisfy a primary need (→ **primäres Bedürfnis**). *Example:* if the need to sleep can be satisfied by a certain condition or locality, a secondary need arises for such circumstances.

Sekundärprozess secondary process.
Conscious mental activity under control of the ego and reality. *cf.* **Primärprozess.**

Selbst self; ego.
Self is the usual translation, e.g. **Selbstanalyse** *self analysis.* "Ego" is a dangerous word used in this sense, although it will occasionally be encountered as a translation, as will **das Ich** for *self.* JUNG considered the "self" to include all parts of the psychic structure. HARTMANN coined the term **Selbstbesetzung** (*self cathexis*), which he distinguished from **Ich-Besetzung** (*ego cathexis*), and defined it as the true contrary of **Objektbesetzung.**

Selbstanklage self-accusation, self-reproach, intropunitiveness.
In everyday language the act of accusing oneself does not necessarily have pathological significance, since it may be justified. In the psychiatric sense, however, this refers to a habit arising from a false sense of guilt.

Selbstaufgabe (des Patienten) self-surrender.

Selbstbeobachtung 1. self observation.
In psychoanalysis this is one of the prime functions of the ego: examination of one's own feelings and behavior. More generally, both terms may refer to observing one's own mental and bodily functions.
2. introspection.
The same as the above but more with regard to reporting the results of such observations in an introspective study.
3. The German expression may also be used in the sense of *hypochondria,* or exaggerating the importance of symptoms, in such constructions as **vermehrte Selbstbeobachtung.**
Ref.: PETERS [11]; Longman [7].

Selbstbestimmungsskala self-rating scale.
A questionnaire or similar device used by a proband or patient in order to assess his own ability, characteristics and attitudes. Employed as an aid to diagnosis.

Selbstentmachtung self-deprivation.

Selbsterfahrung self-awareness, self understanding.
A process in which the patient (or any individual, including the doctor) obtains insight into his attitudes or reactions.

Selbsterhaltungstrieb instinct of self preservation; self-preservation instinct.
The German expression is sometimes written in the plural. *cf.* **Instinkt, → Lebenstrieb, → Trieb.**

Selbstgefühl 1. sense of self.
The feeling of being a distinct individual and having control over one's behavior.
2. sense of identity. Awareness of separate identity.
3. self-concept. Conception and evaluation of one's own qualities and aims. Essentially the same as *self-image.*

Selbsthingabe self-devotion, self dedication (to a cause or ideal); abandon (in the sense of giving oneself over to, or yielding to something, e.g. music).

Selbstwerdung self-actualization.
Full use and exploitation of talent, capacities, potentialities (A. Maslow). Development to maximum self-realization, ideally integrating all needs whether physical, emotional, or intellectual.

Selbstwertgefühle self-esteem.
Some authorities suggest that *self-worth* is the positive evaluation of one's own self that gives rise to the attitude of *self-esteem,* which in turn includes self-acceptance and self-respect.
Ref.: Longman [7].

sensitiver Beziehungswahn (Kretschmer) sensitive delusions of reference. *cf.* **Schlüsselerlebnis.**

sexuelle Aufklärung sex education.
In the formal sense a course of instruction on the reproductive process given in a classroom setting. A more informal approach is often referred to as *instruction in the facts of life.*

sexuelle Erregungskurve sexual-response cycle.
The four stages involved in human orgasm: 1. excitement phase; 2. plateau phase; 3. orgasmic phase; 4. resolution phase.

sexuelle Funktionsstörungen psychosexual disorders.
Impairment of sexual functioning that is caused by psychological rather than organic factors.

Simulant malingerer.

Sinnestäuschung illusion.
Misperceptions of external stimuli, most likely when the general level of sensory stimulation is reduced. It should be distinguished from "delusion" (→ **Wahn**). Also, → **Capgras-Zeichen.**
Ref.: Oxford Textbook of Psychiatry [6], p. 5.

Skala → Schätzskala, → Selbstbestimmungsskala

Skrupel → Beichtskrupel

somatisches Entgegenkommen somatic compliance.
The tendency of a particular organ to express hysterical symptoms. This was Freud's term and is largely identical with symptom choice (→ **Symptomwahl**).

Somatisierung somatization.
Conflicts represented by somatic symptoms. Unlike conversion, the parts or systems involved are innervated by the sympathetic and parasympathetic system; also, a less precise symbolism exists between the conflict and the part affected. *Example:* an ambitious man develops hypertension because his life situation demands that such activity should be curtailed or lessened. Some authorities maintain the term has given way to conversion,

while others use the term *somatization reaction*, which would include psychogenic asthma and peptic ulcers.

Sopor stupor.
The second degree of clouding of consciousness (→ **Bewusstseinstrübung**). The patient is largely unresponsive to all but the most vigorous stimuli, and usually immobile. In brain disease, epilepsy, and toxic states, stupor involves complete unawareness. In catatonic and depressive stupor, however, the patient may be immobile without any loss of consciousness. → **Benommenheit,** → **Koma.**

soziopathische Ulkuskranke tyrannical ulcer-patients.
(*Caveat:* The term "sociopathic" in English connotes stealing, rape, murder etc.) The German expression was the original one in the psychosomatic sense, forming part of the classification of ulcer patients made by OVERBECK and BIEBL. The patients the authors had in mind were those with ego weakness and a tendency towards impulsive outbursts or litigious paranoic behavior, and who fall ill at the faintest suggestion of failure in the sphere of affection.

Spaltung → **Ehespaltung,** → **Persönlichkeitsspaltung.**

Spaltung des Bewusstseins dissociation.
In psychiatric illness, whole areas of mental and physical function may become split off from consciousness. Even in mild forms, conflicts and threatening impulses may be kept apart from the rest of the psyche. The German term covers a broad field and may include such dissociative disorders (DSM-III) as psychogenic fugue and multiple personality. Controversy exists as to whether this is a form of conversion hysteria.
Ref.: Roche Encyclopaedia of Psychiatry [8]; PETERS [11]; Longman [7].

Spannungskopfschmerz tension headache.
Persistent headache, the decisive causes of which are emotional factors. It is a psychosomatic disorder and may be accompanied by insomnia, generalized tension, irritability, and painful contractions of the neck muscles.

Sparsamkeit → **Gesetz der Sparsamkeit.**

Spätdyskinesien → **dyskinetische Spätsyndrome.**

Spätsyndrome → **dyskinetische Spätsyndrome.**

Sperre → **Affektsperre,** → **Bewegungssperre,** → **Gedankensperrung.**

Sprache → **Kunstsprache,** → **Organsprache.**

Sprachverwirrtheit schizophasia.
Unintelligible speech. → **Wortsalat.**

sprunghaftes Denken grasshopper mind.

Stadium des Ausstossens anal expulsive stage.
A phase of the anal period in which pleasure is obtained by expelling feces, or when at an inappropriate time, an expression of defiance against parents.

Stadium des Zurückhaltens anal retentive stage.
A phase of the anal period in which gratification is obtained by retaining feces or defiance against parents is expressed.

Station ward, unit (in a hospital). → **Typ-A-Station,** → **Typ-B-Station.**

Stempeltheorie labeling theory; societal-reaction theory.
The view that classifying or labeling an individual may in itself influence his behavior. The theory found some favor among the antipsychiatrists.

stereotype Bewegungsstörungen stereotyped movement disorders.
Disorders in which involuntary and voluntary repetitive stereotyped movements constitute the main feature. For the various subclasses *cf.* **atypische stereotype Bewegungsstörung,** → **atypischer Tic,** → **Bewegungsstereotypie,** → **chronische motorische Ticstörung,** → **passagerer Tic,** → **Tourette-Störung.**

Stimme(n) voice(s). → **Begleitstimmen.**

Stimmung mood.
Feeling tone, which may be euphoric, despondent, or irritable, and is usually transient. However, ROHRACHER speaks of *moods* when one feeling persists over a long period or actually dominates the various other feelings present. → **Gefühl** (feeling), → **Wahnstimmung.**

Stimmungsveränderungen mood swings.
→ **Verstimmung.**

Stimmungswechsel, Stimmungsumschwung mood swings.
Periodic changes, usually between elation and dejection. In a mild form they are encountered in normally healthy people, but are more severe in neuroses. If greatly exaggerated and persistent they may be symptomatic of manic depression.

Störung disorder, disturbance, defect.
→ **affektive Störungen,** → **Anpassungsstörungen,** → **Bewegungsstörungen,** → **Beziehungsstörung,** → **Einschlafstörungen,** → **Entwicklungsstörung,** → **funktionelle sexuelle Störungen,** → **geistige Entwicklungsstörung,** → **hypersensitive Persönlichkeitsstörung,** → **induzierte paranoide Störung,** → **inhaltliche Denkstörungen,** → **Potenzstörung,** → **psychosomatische Störung,** → **sexuelle Funktionsstörung,** → **Tourette-Störung,** → **Verhaltensstörungen,** → **vorgetäuschte Störungen.**

Störung mit Aufmerksamkeitsdefizit attention-deficit disorder *(DSM-III)*.
A general term for early childhood inattention, lack of concentration, and impulsivity. The two subclasses are attention-deficit disorder with hyperactivity and attention-deficit disorder without hyperactivity.

Strafbedürfnis (FREUD) need for punishment.
Conscious or unconscious need for punishment in order to overcome a sense of guilt. Some authorities relate “accident proneness” to this need.
Ref.: PETERS [11]; Longman [7].

strukturelle Einteilung (seelische Struktur) → Fig. 2.

Studie → **Einzelfallstudie.**

Stumpfheit → **neurotische Stumpfheit.**

Stupor → **Emotionsstupor.**

Sucht addiction.
An extreme state of psychological and sometimes physiological dependence on drugs, alcohol, tobacco, etc. *cf.* **Gewöhnung,** → **Abhängigkeit. Sucht** also has an older meaning – *illness* – that is still retained in such expressions as → **Magersucht.** *cf.* **Betäubungsmittelsucht,** → **Bettsucht,** → **Fressgier,** → **Quälsucht,** → **Zweifelsucht.**

Suchtstoffabhängigkeit drug dependence; substance dependence *(DSM-III)*.
This involves physiological dependence, increased tolerance, and severe withdrawal symptoms. Substances involved include morphine, barbiturates and hallucinogenics. In 1964 the WHO recommended that the term *drug dependence* should include habituation (→ **Gewöhnung**) and addiction (→ **Sucht**) since there was so much overlap.
According to H. COPER, *drug dependence* is produced by continuous administration of a

drug which involves the consumer in a specific behavior leading to further drug intake. The colloquial use of the term refers to psychic dependence, although it is known that in the case of alcohol, opiate or sedative addiction the two other phenomena (tolerance and physical dependence) also exist. The dissociation between tolerance and physical dependence is shown by data on substances like LSD and stimulants.

Ref.: Roche Encyclopaedia [8]; COPER, H.: What is Drug Dependence? Pharmapsychiat. 18 (1985) 323–324.

Sündenbock scapegoat.
The scapegoat mechanism – or more recent "scapegoating" – displaces aggressive impulses and anger onto another person or group. The scapegoat chosen is not responsible for the patient's frustration.

Suizidalität (W. PÖLDINGER) suicidal potential.
The sum of all psychic forces and functions which pave the way to a suicidal act. In a more general sense *suicidal tendency* is used.

symbiontische Psychose symbiontic psychosis.
The term is little used in English, and in German it has a narrower meaning than *folie à deux* (**induzierte paranoide Störung**), being mostly restricted to paranoid schizophrenic patients and the schizoid features they induce in others. Not to be confused with → **symbiotische Psychose.**

symbiotische Psychose symbiotic psychosis.
A rare but serious illness (involving autism) occurring in early childhood characterized by complete dependence on the mother, the chief fear being that of separation. Not to be confused with *folie à deux* (→ **induzierte paranoide Störung**) or → **symbiontische Psychose.**

Symptom → **Grundsymptome,** → **Präsentiersymptom**

Symptome 1. Ranges first-rank symptoms.
KURT SCHNEIDER's method of differential diagnosis for schizophrenia. It is based on the division of symptoms into five categories, which include hallucinations (e.g. écho des pensées → **Gedankenlautwerden**), delusions, changes in thought processes, somatic passivity.

Symptome im Vorstadium symptoms in the prodromal stage (e.g. of several disorders).

Symptomwahl symptom choice.
A term used by ADLER for the "patient's choice" (unconsciously) of one symptom or pattern of symptoms. Sometimes called *choice of a neurosis.*

Syndrom(e) syndromes. → **Abstinenzsyndrom,** → **Adaptationssyndrom,** → **Alkoholentzugssyndrom,** → **dyskinetisches Spätsyndrom,** → **Entziehungserscheinungen,** → **Ganser-Syndrom,** → **KZ-Syndrom,** → **Misshandlungssyndrom,** → **Nachtesser-Syndrom,** → **Psychosyndrom,** → **Schmerzanfälligkeitsyndrom,** psychovegetatives Syndrom (→ **vegetativ**), Tourette-Syndrom (→ **Tourette-Störung**), → **Überlebendensyndrom,** → **Vergewaltigungssyndrom.**

synkretes Denken syncretic thinking.
The first stage in thought processes, in which the child endows all external objects with life in an animistic manner. A broomstick, for example, may be ridden as a horse. It is the stage preceding concrete thinking (*cf.* **konkretes Denken**)

Ref.: Roche Encyclopaedia [8].

syntoner Charakter syntonic character.
A character that is adapted to the individual's surroundings and generally in harmony with the external world. A person possessing this type of character may be called a *syntone.*

System → **Token-Verstärkungssystem.**

Systemtheorie general-systems theory.
A theory seeking to weld the various approaches and types of phenomena studied by science into an entity, human behavior being viewed as a subsystem. It is a form of holistic approach.

Systemtherapie network therapy.
A type of family therapy in which an attempt is made to involve relatives and other persons of reference in the treatment. The object is mainly to keep schizophrenic patients living in the community and avoid rehospitalization.

T

Tachyphylaxie tachyphylaxis.
The decreasing response to a drug. This would appear to be identical with the pharmacological definition of habituation (→ **Gewöhnung**) except that it is generally used in connection with therapy, e.g. the blood-pressure of a patient might continue to rise despite repeated administration of an antihypertensive.

Tagesreste (FREUD) day residues.
Points of contact between dream content and events of the preceding day.

Tasthalluzination tactile hallucination, haptic hallucination.
False perception with regard to the sense of touch. Examples are the feeling of being bitten by insects, sexually abused by unknown persons, or even electrocuted by unseen devices.

Taubheit → **Melodientaubheit.**

Taumel → **Esstaumel.**

täuschen to deceive → **Sinnestäuschung.**

Telefonseelsorge (Germany); **Die dargebotene Hand** (Switzerland); **Kummernummer** (Austria) Samaritans (U.K.).
Voluntary organizations set up for preventing suicide but generally covering crisis intervention for many kinds of acute stress situations. Both the German and the British organizations were originally started under church auspices. The equivalent American organizations include the *telephone support service* and the *crisis team,* but terminology may vary. KIEV favors the term *crisis intervention centers* for the United States.

Ref.: Crisis intervention centers: Oxford Textbook of Psychiatry [6], p. 408.

Tendenz → **Anlehnungstendenzen.**

terminales extrapyramidales Defektsyndrom → **dyskinetische Spätsyndrome.**

themenzentrierte Interaktion interaction-process analysis.
Method developed by BALES for studying intellectual and emotional interactions taking place in group therapy.

Theorie → **Feldtheorie des Verhaltens,** → **Gefühlstheorie,** → **Stempel-Theorie,** → **Systemtheorie.**

Therapie therapy, treatment. → **Beziehungstherapie,** → **Ehepaartherapie,** → **Entspannungstherapie,** → **Erhaltungstherapie,** → **Erkenntnistherapie,** → **Gesprächstherapie,** → **Gestalttherapie,** → **Gestaltungstherapie,** → **Körpertherapie,** → **Kommunikationstherapie,** → **künstlerische Gestaltungstherapie,** → **Kurztherapie (Kurzanalyse),** → **Paartherapie,** → **Systemtherapie,** → **Urschreitherapie, Verhaltenstherapie.**

Thymoleptika thymoleptics.
Tricyclic antidepressants with a primarily mood-elevating effect.

Tic → **Räuspertic.**

Tiefenpsychologie depth psychology.
Approaches focusing on unconscious processes, Freudian psychoanalysis being one of the examples.

Tobsuchtsanfall furor.
An outburst of rage or violent excitation.

Tod → psychogener Tod.

Todeswunsch (FREUD) death wish.
The wish is usually directed towards other persons, (e.g. in oedipal rivalry), but it may be directed inwardly after feelings of guilt.

Token-Verstärkungssystem token economy.
A form of behavior modification. Improvement in behavior is rewarded by tokens that can be exchanged for privileges. Usually employed in a school or hospital setting.

topische Einteilung der Psyche → Fig. 2.

Torschlussjahrzehnten "now-or-never" years.
Derived from **Torschlusspanik**, the last-minute panic before examinations, or a woman's fear of "being left on the shelf".

Totstellreflex feigning death, "playing possum".

Tourette-Störung *Syn.* **Tourette-Syndrom** Tourette's disorder *(DSM-III)*, Tourette's Syndrome.
Involuntary, multiple muscular and vocal tics, the latter developing into words and phrases which may be of obscene content. Once established, the disorder is generally lifelong.

Training → Alphatraining, → psychosomatisches Training.

Tranquiliser; Tranquillanzien tranquilizers; tranquillisers (sometimes in U. K.).
Non-barbiturate sedatives with no antipsychotic effect. → **Neuroleptika.**

Transaktionsanalyse transactional analysis.
A type of psychotherapy focusing on characteristic interactions that reveal internal "ego states" and the "games people play" in social situations. Originator: E. BERNE.

transitorische globale Amnesie transient global amnesia.
Sudden loss of memory generally lasting from 3 to 5 hours. Short-term memory remains intact. The cause is not clear but transient cranial ischemia has been suggested.

Trauerarbeit mourning work; work of mourning; process of mourning; grieving process.
In the Freudian sense the term refers to a phase during which the mourner is able to separate himself from the identity of the deceased. It also describes various phases of emotional change and subsequent progression towards active affective acceptance. The term applies also to such phases passed through after object loss (e.g. loss of health). FREUD described three stages: denial of reality, depression, and adaptation to the new reality. KÜBLER-ROSS listed five: shock and denial; anger; negotiation or bargaining; depression acceptance. **Trauerarbeit schon vor dem Tode, vorzeitige Trauerarbeit** anticipatory mourning. Adaptive processes of parents of relatives during the fatal illness of a patient with terminal illness.
Ref.: 1. GFELLER, A., ASSAL, J.-PH.: The diabetic's subjective experience. In: Folia psychopractica, Editiones Roche, Basle 1980.
2. LUBAN-PLOZZA, B., PÖLDINGER, W.: Psychosomatic Disorders in General Practice. Editiones Roche, Basle 1985.
CRISP, A. H.: Bereavement. Hexagon 'Roche' 14/1 (1986) 14.

Traum → Gefälligkeitstraum.

Traumarbeit (FREUD) dream work.
Transformation of latent dream content into that in which it is experienced by the dreamer (manifest content) (→ **Trauminhalt**). Dream work involves primarily condensation and symbolization, but also displacement, dramatization, and secondary elaboration.

Traumgedanken → Trauminhalt, latenter.

Traumhintergrund dream screen (K. LEWIN).
A screen on which dreams sometimes appear to be projected.

Trauminhalt dream content.
Latenter Trauminhalt latent content. The disguised thoughts and impulses behind symbolic images. **Manifester Trauminhalt** manifest content. The imagery of a dream as experienced by the dreamer.

Traumschuld dream debt.
Lack of REM-sleep (the dream state) which is suppressed by some hypnotics.

Trieb instinct; instinctual drive; drive; urge.
Drive can be used for the primary drives (e.g. sex, hunger and thirst) and the secondary drives, which are acquired – but so can *instinct.* Strictly speaking, *instinct* is more of an inborn behavior pattern, yet the term is frequently employed in translating **Trieb.** *Examples:* **Selbsterhaltungstrieb** instinct of self-preservation. **Todestrieb** death instinct. **Triebiehre** theory of instincts. *Urge* is used in more general senses. *cf.* **Antrieb,** with which there is considerable overlap. Also, → **Instinkt,** → **Geltungstrieb,** → **Geschlechtstrieb,** → **Gesellschaftstrieb,** → **Ichtriebe,** → **Lebenstrieb,** → **Partialtrieb.**

Triebobjekt → **Triebziel.**

Triebziel (FREUD) instinctual aim.
The gratification of an instinct by activity that discharges it. This may be achieved by means of a **Triebobjekt** (the object of an instinct, e.g. food in satisfying hunger).

Trinker → **Betäubungstrinker,** → **Säufer.**

Trinkerheilanstalt, Trinkerheilstätte detoxification center.
This is the usual translation, but whereas the Swiss units tend to restrict themselves to the treatment of alcoholism, those in the United States and some other English-speaking countries also include therapy for drug abuse. Also called a *drying-out center.*

trisomal-dysmorphe Entwicklungsstörung trisomy 21, 21 trisomy.
A condition characterized by the presence of three No. 21 chromosomes in body cells instead of the normal pair. It occurs in most cases of Down's disease.

Trotzverhalten oppositional disorder.
This is *DSM-III* term for a pattern of provocative and defiant behavior aimed chiefly at figures of authority by young people. In less formal descriptions common expressions such as *obstinacy* and *defiant disobedience* would suffice, while "tantrums" in children are only part of the picture.

Trugwahrnehmung → **Sinnestäuschung.**

T-Typ (JAENSCH) T type; tetany type.
This refers to a type of eidetic imagery that persists and assumes a constant form. It is associated with tetany. *cf.* **B-Typ** (definition **2**).

Typ → **A-Typ,** → **B-Typ,** → **C-Typ,** → **Einstellungstypen,** → **Funktionstypen,** → **T-Typ.**

Typ-A-Station Type A general medical ward.
Provides medical care for the acutely ill, with integrated psychosomatic support. Types A and B (→ **Typ-B-Station**) are differentiated in accordance with the recommendations of the → **Enquête-Kommission** on psychiatric and psychosomatic aspects of psychotherapy in the Federal Republic of Germany (1975).
Ref.: KRÖGER, F. et al.: Psychosomatic management of severely ill patients: a patient with lupus erythematosus. Hexagon 'Roche' 13/2 (1985) 24. German (same source): Zum psychosomatischen Umgang mit Schwerkranken: eine Patientin mit lupus erythematodes.

Typ-B-Station Type B psychosomatic clinical ward.
Here psychotherapeutic care is given pride of place (*cf.* **Typ-A-Station**).

Typus → extravertierter Denktypus, → extravertierter Empfindungstypus, → extravertierter Fühltypus, → extravertierter intuitiver Typus, → extravertierter Typus, → introvertierter Denktypus, → introvertierter Empfindungstypus, → introvertierter Fühltypus, → introvertierter intuitiver Typus, → introvertierter Typus.

U

Übelkeit nausea.

Überbeanspruchung overburdening, overstrain.

Überdetermination overdetermination.
In psychoanalysis a multiplicity of drives or motives producing one disorder, dream or behavioral facet.
Ref.: NEEL [10a] p. 185, [10b] S. 238.

Übereinkommen (zwischen Arzt und Patient) tacit collusion, working compromise.
Both terms used by M. BALINT in English publications. The notion is that there may be a danger of the doctor and patient reaching some form of agreement as to treating the symptoms, although this may be ineffective.

Übereinschliessung overinclusiveness (N. CAMERON).
A thought disorder in schizophrenia. An inability to preserve conceptual boundaries, resulting in strange analogies and "wooliness" of thought.

Überflutung (over)flooding. → **Reizüberflutung.**

Über-ich superego.
Conforms to the obligating, restrictive but guiding, rules of society and is thus responsible for conscience and morality.

Überlebendensyndrom → **KZ-Syndrom.**

Überlebensschuld → **KZ-Syndrom.**

übermässige Behütung overprotection.

Übersprungshandlung displacement behavior; displacement activity.
Substitution of one type of behavior by another; particularly in frustration, e.g. scratching the head in perplexity.

Übertragung transference.
The projection of unresolved feelings and attitudes toward parents and important persons of early childhood onto the psychoanalyst.

Übertragungsarbeit the handling of transference (during treatment).

Übertragungsneurose transference neurosis.
Neurotic reactions triggered by the process of transference – early conflicts are revived. Such reactions may replace an original neurosis and provide insight into infantile drives. → **Gegenübertragung.**

Über-uns "super-us".
A term used by HEINROTH, possibly influenced by the collective nature of the force exerted by the superego.

Überwachheit, *Syn.* **Übervigilanz** hypervigilance.
Increased alertness, particularly when due to stimulants, which can develop into nervousness.

Ulkus Ulcer. → **soziopathische Ulkuskranke.**

Umschaltung → **vegetative Umschaltung.**

Umschlag 1. change, swing
E.g. **Umschlag depressiver in manische Zustandsbilder** swing from the depressive to the hypomanic phase.
2. compress; poultice.

unbedingter Reflex unconditioned reflex.
Non-acquired, original response to a stimulus without conditioning.

Unbewusstes unconscious.
In the psychoanalytic sense this is the division of the personality or level of the mind where thoughts and memories are most deeply repressed and can be brought into awareness only when the "censorship" has been overcome. It also harbors id impulses that have never attained verbalization. *cf.* **Vorbewusstes,** → **Unterbewusstes,** → **familiäres Unbewusstes.**

Unfallanfälligkeit accident proneness.
Persons with such chronic susceptibility are sometimes described as having *accident-prone personalities.*

Unfallneurose traumatic neurosis.
Preoccupation with the accident, impairment of memory and concentration. The *DSM-III* term is *posttraumatic stress disorder.*
N.B.: The literal translation, "accident neurosis" is equivalent to "compensation neurosis"; → **Assekurose.**

Ungeschehenmachen undoing.
An attempt, usually ineffective, to make up for feelings of guilt. While the healthy individual will apologize or try to make material amends, an obsessive-compulsive person may attempt to rid himself of guilt by "magical" rites such as excessive hand washing (→ **Waschzwang**). One of the defense mechanisms (→ **Abwehrmechanismen**).

Unlust unpleasure.
The psychoanalytic term describing "ego suffering" and general emotional pain of which a person is conscious when instinctual drives are denied gratification. In a more general sense the German term may be translated by *dislike* or *aversion,* and by *listlessness* when referring to a mood. → **Lebensunlust.**

Unschuldswahn delusions of innocence.
A symptom of prison psychosis in which the prisoner becomes more and more convinced of his innocence.

Unterbewusstes subconscious.
A division of the personality or level of the mind in which thoughts and impulses are fully or partly repressed but may influence conscious thought and concepts. The repressed material may be brought into awareness under certain circumstances, or even spontaneously. The term is thus partly synonymous with the preconscious (→ **Vorbewusstes**) and is not acknowledged by many psychiatrists. → Fig. 2. *cf.* **kollektives Unbewusstes,** → **persönliches Unbewusstes.**

Unterdrückung suppression.
Conscious exclusion of disturbing material from the mind and control over unacceptable feelings and impulses. It should not be confused with "repression" (→ **Verdrängung**). These terms also have biological and genetic connotations, which should be clear from the context.

Unterhaltungstherapie recreational therapy.
Therapy and rehabilitation consisting of pleasurable activities such as excursions, bowling, dancing, hobbies, and social gatherings.

Unterlassungsmanier absence of habitual movements.
The converse of mannerism (→ **Manieriertheit**). The German term includes posturing, mutism, and refusal to eat.

unterstützende Psychotherapie supportive psychotherapy.
Therapy used to help a person through a time-limited crisis without going into the sources or trying to change the basic personality. A variation of "surface therapy" (→ **zudeckende Psychotherapie**) as opposed to

'depth therapy' (→ **aufdeckende Psychotherapie**).

Unterstützung support, reinforcement.

Unzinatusanfall uncinate fit.
An epileptic attack characterized by auras of taste and smell. The hallucinations are usually unpleasant and can precede or follow a dreamy state which may defy description by the patient. The attack indicates a lesion of the temporal lobe in the uncinate region.

Urbild primordial image.
In the Jungian sense the term refers to one of the fundamental archetypes (e.g. mother image) from the collective unconscious that are revived in dreams and twilight states.

Urerlebnis (JANOV) primal event.
→ **Urschreitherapie.**

Urphantasien primal fantasies, unconscious fantasies.
Fanciful conceptions as a substitute for missing facts mostly employed by children, particularly with respect to sexual and reproductive processes. *N.B.:* FOWLER quotes the Oxford English Dictionary in making a distinction between "fantasy" and "phantasy": 'The predominant sense of the former is caprice, whim, fanciful invention, while that of the latter is imagination, visionary notion'.

Urschreitherapie primal therapy; primal-scream therapy (J. JANOV, 1967).
The treatment of neurosis by encouraging the patient to relive basic traumatic events and give vent to them by sobbing, writhing and screaming in an event to discharge painful emotion. The therapy is usually conducted in three phases, briefly: 1. Abstention from stimulants, drugs etc. 2. Re-enactment. 3. Group therapy.

Urszene primal scene.
A child's first real observation between one and two years of age or later imaginary conception of sexual intercourse between parents.

Urverdrängung primary repression, primal repression.
The first phase of repression: unconscious, primordial, or infantile desires that have never become conscious are screened out. In repression proper repressed material has already been in the conscious mind.

V

vagotone Senkung reduction of vagal tone.

vegetativ autonomic, vegetative, visceral.
The English equivalent of this problematic word is usually *autonomic*. There is controversy over the rendering of **psychovegetativ** by "psychoautonomic" (psychophysiological has been suggested), but **das psychovegetative Syndrom** is mainly concerned with autonomic symptoms. The word "vegetative" is best avoided in modern English texts, although it will be found defined as pertaining to those physiological functions concerned with growth, sleep, respiration etc. *Vegetative neurosis* will be found as a translation for **vegetative Neurose** but even this has given way to *visceral neurosis*.

vegetative Umschaltung (J. H. Schultz) changes in autonomic nervous activity.
Changes achieved during autogenic training after practising the "standard" and "meditative" exercises prescribed.
Ref.: Oxford Textbook of Psychiatry [6], p. 614.

Veränderung → Haltungsveränderung.

Verarbeitung working over.
The assimilation of experiences and stimuli, particularly those of early years, into the psychic apparatus (→ **psychischer Apparat**) (Freud) mainly by forming associations. The mental processes implicated modify excitations and prevent possible ill effects from the external discharge of undesirable response. Experiences not integrated into one's own emotional life may have deleterious consequences. → **Angstverarbeitung.**

Verarmungswahn delusion of impoverishment.
A false belief held usually by old or depressive patients that they are on the edge of ruin, that they will accumulate debts and end up poverty-stricken.

Verdichtung condensation.
In the Freudian sense the term refers to the fusion of two or more concepts – or people – into a single item or image, particularly in dreams, but also in neologisms.

Verdrängung repression.
An unconscious defense mechanism which excludes painful experiences and unacceptable impulses from consciousness. It should not be confused with "suppression" (→ **Unterdrückung**). In both languages "repression" has also biochemical, biological and genetic connotations.

Verdrängung des Todes repression of the notion of death. → **Urverdrängung.**

Verfolgungswahn delusion of persecution; persecutory delusion.
An individual's erroneous belief that others are threatening or conspiring against him. This is possibly a projection of the patient's own feelings of guilt to others. The popular term "persecution complex" is best avoided in more formal writing.

Vergewaltigungssyndrom rape-trauma syndrome.
An emotional reaction of rape victims involving nightmares, confusion, shame, fear of sex, repeated washing, and even guilt.
Ref.: Longman [7].

Verhalten → Appetenzverhalten, → Fehlverhalten, → Feldtheorie des Verhaltens, → Trotzverhalten, → Vermeidungsverhalten.

Verhaltungsformung, *Syn.:* **Verhaltensformung** shaping (SKINNER); approximation conditioning.
A therapy based on operant conditioning (→ **operante Konditionierung**), in which behavior is modified step by step. In overcoming phobias, the patient is systematically instructed to do or perceive what he fears.
Ref.: Roche Encyclopaedia [8]; Longman [7].

Verhaltungsstörungen *Syn.:* **Verhaltensstörungen** conduct disorders.
Disorders in social behavior in children and adolescents. *DSM-III* includes five classes: socialized, aggressive; socialized, nonaggressive; undersocialized, aggressive; undersocialized, nonaggressive; atypical.

Verhaltungstherapie, *Syn.:* **Verhaltenstherapie** behavior therapy, behavioral treatment methods, behavior therapies.
Some authorities recommend the plural forms since many techniques exist, including "operant conditioning" (→ **operante Konditionierung**). These methods aim at modifying behavior rather than probing the unconscious or effecting basic changes in the personality.

verharren to persist.
Example: **Wenn sie in ihrem Konflikt verharren** should they become locked in their conflict.

Verinnerlichung 1. inner preoccupation.
Turning away from events in the outside world and total concern with one's own inner world, involving the withdrawal of the libido from its objects. *Egocentricity* has the connotation of being "wrapped up in oneself" or being "the hub of the world" but also that of being selfish.
2. internalization.
The incorporation of the standards and opinions of others, particularly those of the parents, into one's own personality. In this sense it plays a role in superego formation.

Verleugnung denial.
Failing to recognize obvious implications, consequences, or dangers. This is caused by a defense mechanism screening painful or unpleasant events, ideas or wishes. The process takes place at an unconscious level. The terms *disavowal* and *negation* (→ **Verneinung**) are less frequent.

Verlust → **Objektverlust.**

Vermeidungsverhalten avoidance behavior.
Behavior affording escape from painful or unpleasant situations.

Verneinung negation.
A defense mechanism in which the psychoanalyst's interpretation or discovery of repressed material is negated or belittled by the patient. This is held by some authorities to be a form of denial (→ **Verleugnung**).
N.B.: The English term is also used to describe negative constructions in the two-word stage of language development in children, as well as in a general sense.

Verneinungswahn nihilistic delusion; nihilism; delusion of negation.
Pathological conviction of non-existence both of the outside world and parts of the body, usually accompanied by extreme pessimism.

Versagungskomponente component of failure (in therapy).

Verschiebung displacement.
Substitution of one object for another in order to satisfy an instinctual drive. This is a defense mechanism in which, for example, aggressive feeling or violence is directed towards a less threatening object: a man angered by his boss may take it out of his wife or children on his return from work.

Versorgungswünsche → **Hingabebedürfnisse und Versorgungswünsche.**

Verstärkung reinforcement. → **Token-Verstärkungssystem.**

Verstehen understanding; making intelligible.
In the sense in which it was used by JASPERS the term refers to an intuitive grasp of the events in a person's life and their relation to his psychological condition. *cf.* **erklären.**
Ref.: Oxford Textbook of Psychiatry [6], p. 86.

Verstimmung moodiness; ill humor; mood swings; dysphoria.
A vague term in German covering many disturbances or changes in affect. *Mood swings* are more in the direction of **Stimmungsveränderungen. Chronisch-depressive Verstimmung** *constitutional depressive disposition* is rather more specific, and in BLEULER's sense would be the *melancholic mood* of someone who always appears depressed and pessimistic.

Versündigungswahn delusion of sin and guilt.
Pathological conviction of having sinned or being responsible for many untoward events.

Verwirrtheit confusion. → **Sprachverwirrtheit.**

Verworrenheit thought derailment; thought disorganization; knight's move.
A loosening of associations with no logical relationship between the various topics entered upon.
Ref.: Oxford Textbook of Psychiatry [6], p. 11; PETERS [11].

Vitalangst fear for one's life.
This fear stems from within the body and has a signal function; the anxiety a patient has on experiencing a sudden heart attack causes him to keep still and seek medical aid. Once such aid has been granted, however, this fear may have a negative influence.

vitale Traurigkeit vital sadness.
Encountered in cases of endogenous depression. Incapacity to derive pleasure from life, accompanied by sluggishness and listlessness. It might have been better to use the word *devitalized*, since the term is employed to describe a *loss* of vital impulses and feelings.

Vollkommenheitswahn perfectionism.
A striving for standards that are usually higher than the situation demands. The tasks on hand are sometimes never terminated. The word **Wahn** is really out of place here, and the current German expression is **Perfektionismus.**

Vorbeireden talking past the point, "beating around the bush" (U.S.), "beating about the bush" (U.K.).
The patient never quite reaches the point. Sometimes associated with Ganser's syndrome, → **Gefängnispsychose.**
Ref.: Oxford Textbook of Psychiatry [6], p. 11; Longman [7], p. 789.

Vorbewusstes preconscious.
In psychoanalysis the preconscious is sometimes defined as a division of the personality and sometimes as a level of consciousness from which ideas, memories, and impulses can readily be brought to the conscious mind. → Fig. 2.

vorgetäuschte Störungen factitious disorders.
The simulation of physical or emotional symptoms. It is intentional but has a psychological cause. *DSM-III* thus differentiates such disorders from malingering in which no psychological cause exists.

Vorlust forepleasure.
Pleasure obtained by exciting erogenous zones prior to sexual intercourse; may lead to end pleasure after puberty (→ **Endlust**). Similar to "foreplay", except that this is sometimes regarded as the first stage of sexual

response and accompanied by physical effects.

Vorsatzformel autosuggestive recitation or slogan.
The method is known as "couéism" and consists of giving suggestions to oneself to improve morale or promote recovery. Evolved from EMILE COUÉ.

Vorstadium prodromal stage of a disorder.

Vorstellung thought, idea. → **Zwangsvorstellung.**

W

Wachanfall nocturnal hemiplegia; sleep paralysis.
Inability to move or speak during brief periods while mentally alert, usually when falling to sleep. Frequently associated with narcolepsy.

Wach-Schlaf-Rhythmus sleep-wake cycle. → **Schlaf-Wach-Rhythmus.**

Wachzustand waking state, W-state. → **orthodoxer Schlaf.**

Wahl → **Neurosenwahl,** → **Symptomwahl.**

Wahn delusion; mania; madness (lay term).
A delusion is a *belief* or conviction that is held despite evidence to the contrary. *Mania* is a state of overexcitement, agitation and hyperactivity. In English there are both *religious delusions* and *religious mania.* → **Sinnestäuschung, Capgras-Zeichen,** → **Beachtungswahn,** → **Beziehungswahn,** → **Begnadigungswahn,** → **Berufungswahn,** → **Eifersuchtswahn,** → **Größenwahn** → **Kontaktwahn,** → **Krankheitswahn,** → **Liebeswahn,** → **metaphorischer Wahn,** → **Offenbarungswahn,** → **Primärwahn,** → **Querulantenwahn,** → **Unschuldswahn,** → **Verarmungswahn,** → **Verneinungswahn,** → **Versündigungswahn, Vollkommenheitswahn.**

Wahnstimmung delusional mood.
Usually a foreboding that some sinister event is about to take place. The term has been criticized. The essence is that delusions generally occur before the feeling, while here the feeling occurs first.
Ref.: Oxford Textbook of Psychiatry [6], p. 15.

Wahrnehmung perception.
Awareness via the senses and gaining a meaningful picture of our surroundings by recognition and discrimination. → **außersinnliche Wahrnehmung.** → **Trugwahrnehmung.**

Wahrnehmung, bewusste → **Apperzeption.**

Wahrnehmungsgegenstand percept.
The product and modification of perception as experienced.

Wandlungen transformations.
Example: **Wandlungen und Symbole der Libido** 'Study of the Transformations and Symbolisms of the Libido' – a translation of part of C. G. JUNG's *Jahrbuch* by B. M. HINKLE.

Waschzwang compusive handwashing. ablutomania.
An obsessive-compulsive disorder in which patients repeatedly wash their hands. While this may be associated with fear of dirt and germs, it may also constitute a ritual against feelings of guilt. The alternative term *ablutomania* may be misleading in that persons with other manias may actually enjoy carrying out their impulsive act, e.g. the pyromaniac, whereas those suffering from compulsive handwashing gain no pleasure and are frequently under considerable stress.

Wechsel change, exchange, shift.
→ **Rollenwechsel,** → **Stimmungswechsel.**

Wechselwirkung interaction.
Relationships between two or more persons or groups that exert reciprocal effects and influence. Hence *interaction-process analysis* **(themenzentrierte Interaktion).**

Weglaufen running away, evasion. → **psychogenes Weglaufen.**

Weichteilrheumatismus soft tissue rheumatism.
Now the term preferred to "extra-articular rheumatism".

Weitschweifigkeit divagation.
Rambling and digression in either speech or thought. **Weitschweifiges Denken** refers to a loose form of thought that is overburdened with unnecessary detail and constantly digresses to other topics. This occurs in elderly people and in patients with cerebral sclerosis, but it may be a characteristic of other persons. It comes very close to *tangential thinking* in which there are interruptions in the train of thought as well as the tendency of "fly off at a tangent". In its extreme form it may be a symptom of schizophrenia.

Werdung → Selbstwerdung.

Werkstätte → beschützende Werkstätte.

Wesensänderung personality change.
This is the usual translation, though *irreversible personality change* would in most cases be nearer to the German term, which is defined as arising from varied causes ranging from emotional and organic trauma to hormonal disorders and schizophrenia.

wiederaufleben lassen redintegrate; reintegrate; rearouse.
Experiences in later life may *redintegrate* earlier problems if they involved similar patterns or trauma. *Redintegration* is also the organization of mental processes after disorganization by a psychosis and the recollection of memories from cues.
Ref.: NEEL [10a] S. 236, [10b] p. 181; Longman [7].

Wiederaufnahme re-uptake;
Example: neuronal re-uptake of transmitter (primarily after release).

Wiederholungszwang repetition-compulsion.
Repetition of behavior patterns serving no useful or pleasurable purpose. The condition is seen in many types of neurosis. FREUD used the term to describe an unconscious need to reenact early traumas in an attempt to overcome them.

Wille zur Macht → Machtstreben.

Willenlosigkeit abulia (sometimes aboulia).
A pathological inability to make decisions or take any initiative. It is encountered in schizophrenia and occasionally in depression or neuroses.

Wirklichkeitsentfremdung feelings of unreality.
If this sensation relates to the persons himself feeling unreal or changed one speaks of *depersonalization*. Should such feelings relate to surroundings, however, the term is *derealization*. If extreme, it may be a symptom of schizophrenia.

Wissen → Erfahrungswissen.

Wochenbettdepression postpartum depression; puerperal depression.
Depressive disorders usually beginning after the first two weeks of the puerperium. Tiredness, irritability, and anxiety are more prominent than depressive mood change. Phobic symptoms may also be present.
Ref.: Oxford Textbook of Psychiatry [6], p. 392.

Wochenbettpsychose postpartum psychosis, puerperal psychosis.
A now rare psychosis occurring within six weeks after delivery. It is usually schizophrenic and sometimes depressive in character. Such psychosis is thought to be associated with the stresses of the puerperium, and hormonal changes may act as precipitants. The condition may also be aggravated by preexisting personality defects and maladjustments.

Wollen volition.
The voluntary choice of a course of action without direct external influence.

Wonnesaugen → **Daumenlutschen.**

Wortagglutination; *Syn.* **Wortverklebung** contamination.
In psychiatry this is the amalgamation of two words to form another of doubtful sense. A form of neologism. Although sometimes pathological, it is sometimes used in humor. The usual German expression is **Kontamination.**

Wortsalat word salad, word hash, jargon aphasia.
An incoherent mixture of words or phrases commonly associated with schizophrenia.

Wortzauber incantation; word spells.
A form of magical thinking existing among primitive peoples and schizophrenics that words can control certain events. Also present unconsciously in civilized and healthy people, for example in utterances such as "talk of the devil and he will appear".

Wunsch wish, desire. → **Todeswunsch.**

Z

Zählzwang arithmomania, obsessive-compulsive impulse to count.

Zärtlichkeitsspiele foreplay (in a sexual sense).

Zeitbewusstseinsstörung time distortion.
A form of perceptual distortion in which time appears either to pass very slowly or exceedingly fast. The disturbance occurs in altered states of consciousness.

Zelle → **Isolierzelle.**

Zeremoniell ritual. → **Einschlafzeremoniell,** → **Zwangszeremoniell.**

Zerrüttung 1. (des Geistes) derangement **2.** (der Ehe) break-up; **familiäre Zerrüttung** broken home.

Ziel aim, goal, target. → **Triebziel.**

Zielsymptome target symptoms.

Zopfabschneiden braid-cutting.
The fetish of clipping a pigtail or tress of hair from a woman. Freud related it to symbolic castration.

zudeckende Psychotherapie surface therapy; non-analytical techniques.
Psychotherapeutic techniques in which conflicts are not made conscious. These include autogenic training and counseling. For practical reasons (time), such methods are more frequent than uncovering techniques (→ **aufdeckende Psychotherapie**).

Zurechnungsunfähigkeit incompetency (to stand trial).
In common law the "incompetency plea" is invoked when a defendant is not legally responsible for his or her actions owing to mental disease.

zurückhalten to keep back, to retain. → **Stadium des Zurückhaltens.**

Zusammenschrecken startle reaction.
Rapid response to sudden, unexpected stimulus such as noise or danger. The usual signs are flexion of the trunk and extremities, increased respiration and alertness.

Zustand → **Geisteszustand,** → **Wachzustand.**

Zwang 1. compulsion.
The uncontrollable and irrational (subjective) pressure to perform a stereotyped act. Some authors distinguish between *compulsion* and *impulse.* The latter can be experienced as pleasurable, but not compulsion. *cf.* **Waschzwang** and the ensuing example.
2. obsessive-compulsion in the sense of **Zwangserscheinungen**.
Obsession refers to ideas forcibly intruding on the consciousness, e.g. in "obsessive fantasy", while *compulsion* involves affective components, acts, and drives. Despite these generalizations, there appears to be some overlap in English usage: *anankastic personality disorder* is found in *ICD-9* for *obsessional personality disorder,* but *DSM-III* prefers *compulsive personality* to either of these terms.
3. While *compulsion* and *obsession* are the usual translations in psychological contexts, **Zwang** may be rendered quite differently in other fields, e.g. **Zwangsernährung** force feeding or forced feeding. → **Gegenzwang,** → **Geständniszwang,** → **Grübelzwang,** → **Kontrollzwang.**

Zwangsantrieb obsessive impulse.
An irresistible urge to perform an offensive act that is against one's will.

Zwangsbefürchtungen *Syn.:* **Phobien** (a Germanization). → Appendix pp. 93–95.

Zwangseinweisung compulsory admission (to a psychiatric hospital).
Commitment is the usual expression in English, meaning that the patient is to be confined by court order, frequently against his will.

Zwangserbrechen recurrent involuntary vomiting; psychogenic vomiting.
Ref.: Oxford Textbook of Psychiatry [6], p. 370.

Zwangsjacke camisole; straitjacket

Zwangslachen compulsive laughter.
Uncontrollable laughter for no reason. It is a frequent symptom in the disorganized type of schizophrenia. → **Lachkrampf.**

Zwangsneurose obsessive-compulsive neurosis; obsessive-compulsive disorder *(DSM-III);* anankastic neurosis *(ICD-9).*
The original German expression stems from Freud. The symptoms represent a compromise between wish-fulfillment drives (censored by the superego) and vicarious gratifications. This results in ambivalence. Obsessive-compulsive disorders are defined by *ICD-9* as a state in which "the outstanding symptom is a feeling of subjective compulsion – which must be resisted – to carry out some action, to dwell on an idea, to recall an experience, or to ruminate on an abstract topic . . .". The definition goes on to say that the urge is recognized as alien to the personality but as coming from within the self.
Ref.: Oxford Textbook of Psychiatry [6], p. 163; Glossary of Mental Disorders (WHO) [9], p. 36; Peters [11].

Zwangsvorstellung obsession; obsessional thought.
The second English term is less used, but probably nearer to the German since "obsession" may include not only ideas, memories and images that intrude on the consciousness against the will, but also impulses.

Zwangszeremoniell obsessional rituals.
Repeated, senseless, routines such as laying out clothes in a specific, complicated manner before being able to dress.

Zweifelsucht doubting mania; obsessional doubt.
Persistent doubt as to whether a task has been properly completed. A common symptom of obsessive-compulsive disorder.

Zweizügelabhängigkeit dependence on a combination of substances.
Dependency on both stimulants and sedatives; e.g. amphetamines taken in the morning may incur a need for barbiturates in the evening, and vice-versa. This applies mainly to the second category listed in *DSM-III:* dependence on combination of substances, excluding opioids and alcohol.

zwischenmenschlicher Konflikt interpsychic conflict.
Conflict arising within individuals from external sources, e.g. noise made by neighbors. A better term would probably be **sozialer Konflikt** in German, and *psychosocial conflict* in English. → **innerseelischer Konflikt.**

Appendix

Tabelle weniger bekannter Phobien
Table of lesser-known phobias

Classical term	Krankhafte Angst	Morbid fear
Achluophobia	vor der Dunkelheit	of darkness
Acrophobia	vor der Höhe	of heights
Aerophobia	vor dem Durchzug und vor Gas	of draughts, gases
Agyiophobia	vor Strassen	of the street
Aichmophobia	vor spitzen Gegenständen	of sharp objects
Ailurophobia	vor Katzen	of cats
Amatophobia	vor Staub	of dust
Amaxophobia	in einem Fahrzeug zu sein	of being in a vehicle
Anemophobia	vor dem Wind	of wind
Anginophobia	vor dem Ersticken	of suffocation
Apeirophobia	vor dem Unendlichen	of the infinite
Apiphobia	vor Bienen	of bees
Arachneophobia	vor Spinnen	of spiders
Astraphobia	vor Gewitter	of thunderstorms
Astrophobia	vor Sternen	of stars
Basiphobia	vor dem Laufen	of walking
Basophobia	vor dem Aufrechtstehen	of standing erect
Bathophobia	vor der Tiefe	of depths
Belonephobia	vor Nadeln	of needles
Bromidrosiphobia	vor (eigenem) Körpergeruch	of (personal) body odor
Brontophobia	vor dem Donner	of thunder
Cheimaphobia	vor der Kälte	of the cold
Cherophobia	vor der Fröhlichkeit	of gaiety
Chionophobia	vor Schnee	of snow
Chrematophobia	vor Geld	of money
Climacophobia	vor Treppen	of stairs
Cypri(do)phobia	vor Geschlechtskrankheiten	of venereal diseases
Daemonophobia	vor Dämonen	of demons
Demophobia	vor Menschenmengen	of crowds
Dikephobia	vor der Justiz	of justice
Eisoptrophobia	vor Spiegeln	of mirrors
Eosophobia	vor der Morgendämmerung	of dawn

Classical term	Krankhafte Angst	Morbid fear
Erythrophobia	vor Rot, Errötung, und Blut	of red, blushing, and blood
Galeophobia = ailurophobia = Gatophobia	vor Katzen	of cats
Gephyrophobia	vor Brücken	of bridges
Hamartophobia	vor Sünden und Fehlern	of sin, errors
Haphephobia = Haptephobia	vor dem Berührtwerden	of being touched
Harpaxophobia	vor Dieben	of thieves
Hedonophobia	vor dem Vergnügen	of pleasure
Hierophobia	vor heiligen oder religiösen Gegenständen	of sacred or religious things
Hodophobia	vor Reisen	of travel
Homilophobia	vor Predigten	of sermons
Hydrophobia	vor Wasser	of water
Hydrophobophobia	vor der Hydrophobie oder Tollwut	of hydrophobia or of rabies
Hylephobia	vor dem Materialismus	of materialism
(H)ylophobia	vor Wäldern	of forests
Hypengyophobia	vor der Verantwortung	of responsibility
Hypsophobia = acrophobia	vor der Höhe	of heights
Iophobia	vor Gift	of poison
Kaino(to)phobia	vor dem Neuen	of new things
Kakorrhaphiophobia	vor dem Versagen	of failure
Kenophobia	vor leeren Flächen	of large open spaces
Kopophobia	vor der Ermüdung	of fatigue
Levophobia	vor Gegenständen auf der linken Seite	of objects on the left side
Logophobia	vor (öffentlichem) Sprechen	of (public) speaking
Lyssophobia	verrückt zu werden oder vor der Tollwut	of becoming insane, or of rabies
Molysophobia	vor der Ansteckung	of contamination
Musophobia	vor Mäusen	of mice
Mysophobia	vor der Ansteckung von Bakterien oder Schmutz (Vorstufe von **Waschzwang** q.v.)	of contamination by germs or dirt (precursor to compulsive handwashing)
Ochlophobia = demophobia	vor Menschenmengen	of crowds
Ombrophobia	vor Regen	of rain

Classical term	Krankhafte Angst	Morbid fear
Osphresiophobia	vor Gerüchen	of odours
Paralipophobia	seine Pflichten zu vernachlässigen	of neglecting obligations
Peccatiphobia = hamartophobia	zu sündigen	of sinning
Peniaphobia	vor der Armut	of poverty
Phasmophobia	vor Geistern	of ghosts
Phobophobia = maniaphobia	vor der Furcht, dem Irrsin	of fearing, of insanity
Pnigophobia = anginophobia	vor dem Ersticken	of suffocation
Potamophobia	vor Gewässern	of rivers
Psychrophobia = cheimaphobia	vor der Kälte	of the cold
Pteronophobia	vor Federn	of feathers
Rhypophobia	vor dem Schmutz	of filth
Scopophobia =	gesehen zu werden;	of being seen;
Scoptophobia	sich lächerlich zu machen	of being ridiculous
Scotophobia = achluophobia	vor der Dunkelheit	of darkness
Siderodromophobia	vor der Eisenbahn	of railway travel
Spectrophobia = eisoptrophobia	vor Spiegeln	of mirrors
Stygiophobia	vor der Hölle	of hell
Tredecaphobia = Triskaidekaphobia	vor der Zahl 13	of the number 13
Uranophobia	vor dem Himmel	of heaven
Zelophobia	vor der Eifersucht	of jealousy

Personal Notes